PRAISE FOR *TO REPAIR THE WORLD*

"Whenever there is a need, Paul is the first guy out the door. His humility is legendary and one hundred percent genuine. Medical students all over the world have told me they entered our shared profession because of Dr. Paul Farmer. Now, it is time for the rest of the planet to be inspired, and in these pages they learn what it takes to repair the world."

—Sanjay Gupta, Chief Medical Correspondent at CNN and Associate Chief of Neurosurgery at Emory University School of Medicine

"Paul Farmer is the most compelling voice for justice in a generation. In this volume are the stories and insights that have helped thousands of students imagine—and fight for—a better world. Read this to be inspired. Read this to learn. Most importantly, when you're done, give this book to a friend and join the movement for health equity."

—Jonny Dorsey, cofounder of FACE AIDS and Global Health Corps

"This is a bold read by a humble visionary. For those who care about humanity, this is a handbook for the heart."

—Byron Pitts, Chief National Correspondent, CBS Evening News

"Here is Paul at those special moments when we want and need a moral exemplar, calling us to do what good we can for those who have nothing, who are broken, who are left behind, who are sick and disabled, who need to be accompanied, and whose betterment betters us."

—Arthur Kleinman, Esther and Sidney Rabb Professor of Anthropology at Harvard University

"Paul Farmer has a knack for persuading an audience to participate in his lectures, whether aloud or in silence. The liveliness of his talks comes in part from his delivery, but also from the qualities of the lectures themselves: the freshness of their ideas, their wit, and their passion. And these, thankfully, are qualities that this collection preserves."

—Tracy Kidder, Pulitzer Prize–winning author of *The Soul of a New Machine, Among Schoolchildren, Mountains Beyond Mountains,* and other titles

"This book inspires us all—students, teachers, artists, politicians, businesspeople— to use our life's work as a source of good. Paul Farmer exposes all the excuses we make for ourselves not to make this world a better place."

—Régine Chassagne, founding member of Arcade Fire

To Repair the World

The publisher gratefully acknowledges the generous support of the Anne G. Lipow Endowment Fund for Social Justice and Human Rights of the University of California Press Foundation, which was established by Stephen M. Silberstein

To Repair the World

*Paul Farmer
Speaks to the Next Generation*

Edited by Jonathan Weigel

With a foreword by President Bill Clinton

UNIVERSITY OF CALIFORNIA PRESS

University of California Press, one of the most distinguished university presses in the United States, enriches lives around the world by advancing scholarship in the humanities, social sciences, and natural sciences. Its activities are supported by the UC Press Foundation and by philanthropic contributions from individuals and institutions. For more information, visit www.ucpress.edu.

University of California Press
Oakland, California

First Paperback Printing 2019

Library of Congress Cataloging-in-Publication Data
Farmer, Paul, 1959–
    [Speeches. Selections]
    To repair the world : Paul Farmer speaks to the next generation /
edited by
Jonathan Weigel ; foreword by President Bill Clinton.
        pages   cm
    ISBN 978-0-520-27597-3 (hardback); 978-0-520-32115-1 (pbk. : alk. paper)
    1. Public health—Social aspects.   2. Public welfare.   3. Public
health administration.   4. Public health—Citizen participation.
5. Public health—Addresses   I. Weigel, Jonathan, 1986–   II. Title.
RA418.F36   2013
362.1—dc23   2013002004

Manufactured in the United States

21   20   19
10   9   8   7   6   5   4   3   2   1

To Jennie Block, with deep gratitude
for her accompaniment over the years

P.F.

CALIFORNIA SERIES
IN PUBLIC ANTHROPOLOGY

The California Series in Public Anthropology
emphasizes the anthropologist's role as an engaged
intellectual. It continues anthropology's commitment
to being an ethnographic witness, to describing, in
human terms, how life is lived beyond the borders
of many readers' experiences. But it also adds a
commitment, through ethnography, to reframing
the terms of public debate—transforming received,
accepted understandings of social issues with new
insights, new framings.

Series Editor:
Robert Borofsky (Hawaii Pacific University)

Contributing Editors:
Philippe Bourgois (University of Pennsylvania),
Paul Farmer (Partners In Health),
Alex Hinton (Rutgers University),
Carolyn Nordstrom (University of Notre Dame), and
Nancy Scheper-Hughes (UC Berkeley)

University of California Press Editor:
Naomi Schneider

Volume 29. To Repair the World:
Paul Farmer Speaks to the Next Generation

CONTENTS

FOREWORD

PRESIDENT BILL CLINTON

I've learned that in addressing any country's—and the world's—most pressing challenges, competition can almost always be fruitful. This shouldn't be surprising; think of how often we hear calls for competitiveness in business, or how we value the achievements of a superior jazz musician or athlete. But while good policy will draw on this tension among competitors, to solve the great social problems before us, from climate change to pandemic disease, we know we need to turn from competition to cooperation and partnership. This is especially true when these problems afflict the poor and marginalized, as they disproportionally do. It's this unfair distribution of the world's hardships that Paul Farmer has spent thirty years addressing tirelessly as a physician, a teacher, and an increasingly influential policy voice. It was Paul's belief in the power of cooperation, across lines of nationality, class, language, and race, that led him to found Partners In Health while still a student at Harvard Medical School. That abiding belief and a call for renewed engagement from young Americans lie at the heart of the speeches collected here in *To Repair the World.* The truth is I was the last in my family to get to know Paul. When Hillary was First Lady, she brought him to the White House to discuss one of the gravest new health problems facing some regions of the world: highly drug-resistant tuberculosis. Paul had been tackling this disease in Haiti, Peru, and Russia, not only working to cure patients but also sounding the alarm that this is not a problem that will go away and will only grow with inaction—a prediction, like many Paul made in the nineties, that has unfortunately come to pass. When I read a *New Yorker* profile of Paul in 2000, I immediately called Chelsea to draw him to her attention. She told me she already knew him and said something I never forgot. He is, she told me, "our generation's Albert Schweitzer."

Since then I've been lucky enough to work closely with Paul for more than a decade in Haiti and also in settings as far-flung as Rwanda and Malawi. He has been not only one of my closest advisers regarding global health but also one of those rare people who, along with his Partners In Health team, is actually on the ground providing health care. Paul is never content merely to point out and deplore problems. Instead, he and his colleagues go to work on solving them, which is why, from South America to Siberia, Partners In Health is still involved in caring for some of the most marginalized people suffering with tuberculosis, AIDS, and other diseases of the poor.

AIDS was a major challenge for my administration and for anyone who, like Paul, was working as a physician in settings of poverty, inequality, and disruption. During my time in office we doubled the amount of funding going into AIDS research, focusing on building up a portfolio of solutions reaching from basic science to clinical trials. All of us were rewarded for this investment when the number of effective drugs went from two in 1992 to more than two dozen in 2000. But rolling these discoveries and advances out to the rest of the world was, and remains, a monumental task, and one that led to Paul's second and more consequential trip to the White House, this time under a new administration.

When historians look back on George W. Bush's presidency, I'm inclined to think that they will agree with me that his leading contribution was PEPFAR, the President's Emergency Plan for AIDS Relief. What is less known is Paul's role in taking it from a concept—and what sounded to many like a pipe dream—to reality. When the Bush Administration began its due diligence on the draft policy, it called in physicians, including Paul and PIH, who were having remarkable success treating AIDS patients with antiretroviral therapy in rural Cange, Haiti. It put Cange on the policy map, earning a squatter settlement an improbable spot in the long history of fighting infectious diseases. It also set the stage for PEPFAR's success. PEPFAR has already saved millions of lives and is one of the reasons that PIH cofounder Dr. Jim Yong Kim went on to the World Health Organization to head up the "3 by 5" Initiative, seeking to put three million people on treatment by 2005.

When I left office, the prospect of millions of Africans on therapy was still a dream. One of the first things I did in 2002 was to start the Clinton HIV/AIDS Initiative, headed by Ira Magaziner. The first person I consulted was Paul, hard at work in rural Haiti. A few years later, understanding all too well that increased funding and decreased drug prices would not solve what Paul and Dr. Kim called "the delivery gap," we launched, jointly with PIH and local ministries of health, the Rural Africa

Initiative. This was designed to build up health care capacity in rural areas of Rwanda, Malawi, Lesotho, and Haiti, since AIDS is only one of many health problems in these settings. In Rwanda, PIH has worked closely with the Ministry of Health and with my foundation to expand primary care to a substantial fraction of that beautiful country's population. It's not by accident that last year Rwanda became one of the first two countries in sub-Saharan Africa to reach something close to universal access to AIDS therapy. The other country was wealthier Botswana. Rwanda is also the only country in the region on track to meet the Millennium Development Goals.

As AIDS, malaria, and tuberculosis take fewer lives and as life expectancy increases, new problems emerge. I was there not a year ago to cut the ribbon on what is probably rural Africa's first cancer treatment center, which the Ministry of Health opened with the help of many partners, including PIH and the Harvard hospitals where Paul works when not abroad. It is certainly one of the most lovely hospitals I have ever seen and stands as evidence of the potential that arises from the best kind of cooperation, from bringing together the skills and resources of the developed and developing worlds, of public and private entities, and of many countries, including the United States and Haiti.

In 2004, Haiti was disrupted by yet another coup, which made it difficult for me to work there, since CHAI only works in countries where we can partner with governments to have the greatest impact. As Paul and his family headed off to Rwanda, the PIH team continued its work in Haiti, expanding its public-private partnership across the country, from the Dominican border to the coast. A few years later, Paul called me from the drowned city of Gonaïves, hammered by four hurricanes in one month, asking what I might be able to do to help. Within a few months, the Secretary General of the United Nations, Ban Ki-moon, named me the United Nations Special Envoy for Haiti. The idea was to bring in new partners to support Haitian businesses and entrepreneurs, since whatever one's political leanings, all agreed that it was Haiti's stagnant economy that had created an environment conducive to the kind of health problems Paul had seen for decades and also made the country particularly vulnerable to the impact of natural disasters. In the fall of 2009, Paul became my volunteer deputy and turned some of his talents and attention to improving policy around foreign aid for Haiti.

Then came the earthquake of January 12, 2010.

Paul and his family had just left Haiti, and we spoke that evening. I asked him to come immediately to the UN where I addressed the General Assembly: Haiti urgently needed the support of the world and also a sound plan for relief and reconstruction. With Hillary's help, we had Paul back in Haiti within a day, at first serving as a physician to the staggering number of earthquake victims and later as a policy expert to help Haiti "build back better." He has described this experience in another book, *Haiti After the Earthquake,* which vividly tells the story of that terrible time. The seismic disaster was followed by an epidemic of cholera, the first to affect Haiti in recorded memory, to which PIH brought vital scientific expertise, medical care, and investment in oral vaccines.

The speeches included in this book cover all these topics and many more, and they also reflect Paul's insistence as a lifelong teacher that young Americans—especially those privileged enough to attend our best universities and medical schools and who later move into the kind of roles he has pioneered—embrace his vision of a world of shared opportunity and shared responsibility. I've often said in print and in person that the explosion of private citizens doing public good is the most meaningful trend of our times, which is why I strongly believe Paul's efforts should be recognized by a Nobel Prize, to inspire other bright young men and women to follow in his footsteps.

Paul's personal strengths—his commitment to justice, his determination to fight on behalf of the poor, his tenacity in following up with patients and families, his dogged focus on making good policies and seeing them through to implementation, and his immense reservoir of optimism—make him the ideal teacher of how to change the way we see the world and how each of us can do the kinds of things he does in our local communities or halfway around the world. The essence of Paul Farmer's inspiration is here in these pages, as it is in every chapter of his life so far and will be in the days and years to come.

INTRODUCTION

JONATHAN WEIGEL

Anyone who has heard Dr. Paul Farmer speak knows the pull of his stories, the speed of his wit, and the force of his vision. When he describes the work of Partners In Health (PIH) in Haiti or Rwanda or Russia, we can't suppress the feeling that he's figured out what it means to do the right thing, to make the world a better place. It's inspiring. It's also uncomfortable because that right thing rarely resembles what we do every day. He makes us face poverty and injustice, which most of the time we are content to ignore. He makes us pay attention to people suffering, sometimes dying, from diseases for which we could pick up treatments in a corner pharmacy. We can't help asking ourselves what we, each of us, might do to help lessen such towering inequity.

This book is a collection of some of Paul's most memorable speeches, at university graduations and other public venues. Unlike many of his writings in clinical medicine, global public health, and anthropology, these are written principally for a general audience and especially for young people considering what path to tread in the years that await them.[1] We hope this volume will make Paul's vision of social justice and radical solidarity with the world's poor accessible to readers from all walks of life.

I. "YOU GUYS ARE MY HEROES"

I met Paul when he came to speak at my high school in 2005. We were excited to meet a person of such stature and were prepared to be impressed and inspired. But we were not at all prepared for how funny he was, how he seemed to look each of us straight in the eye with the full weight of his big personality, how he got away with being so sincere and so passionate, how he made complicated ideas accessible and exciting, how he made us feel like peers, partners, coconspirators.

His presentation detailed PIH's efforts to provide AIDS treatment in an impoverished squatter settlement in rural Haiti. I was moved and inspired and more than a little uncomfortable. My planner was filled with biology classes, piano lessons, cross-country practice, and other things wholly alien to the hardscrabble life Paul described in Haiti. My main goal was getting into college. Should I harness the good fortune of my privileged upbringing to work on behalf of those born in less fortunate circumstances thousands of miles away?

At one point, someone asked him an awkward, perhaps impertinent question: what is it like to be a hero? "Well," he said without hesitation, "you guys are my heroes," referring to all of us packed in the auditorium, which was overflowing into the hall. "In fact, you're my retirement plan." Maybe it sounds trite now, but we could tell he meant it. Paul Farmer was in high demand as a speaker nationally and internationally; he wouldn't have made the effort to come to our high school if he didn't believe that students had a key role to play in the movement for global health equity.

This realization—that students were protagonists in Paul Farmer's vision of a more humane world—became clearer when I arrived at Harvard College a year later. In between running a department at the Medical School, a division at Brigham and Women's Hospital, a center at the School of Public Health, and of course continuing the work and expansion of Partners In Health, Paul and PIH cofounder Dr. Jim Yong Kim made time to advise a global health student group I joined. Sometimes they asked us to organize events; sometimes they solicited our advice about new courses they were developing; always they were eager to learn how to draw more students toward global health. The point is that they took us seriously. We weren't just pesky students asking for good grades and recommendation letters (though we were all that, too); we were partners in something big and important.

My senior year, Paul, Jim, and Dr. Arthur Kleinman, who had taught Paul and Jim as doctoral students, offered a new class.[2] It was just what we had asked for: a comprehensive introduction to global health. The professors had lines out the door every week during office hours, but they stuck around until all of our questions had been answered. (I would later learn that, much to the bewilderment and occasional consternation of his staff, Paul regularly delayed "real" meetings and flights to stay in office hours until we students had had our fill.)

I started working on Paul's team at Partners In Health a year later. Orientation consisted of a one-line Blackberry-typed email from the doctor himself: "It's going to be a baptism by fire." No one could have said it better. Paul is all in, all the time. And everyone who works with him feels inspired—compelled—to do the same. I soon found myself helping Paul prepare for lectures, editing books and articles, and accompanying Paul as he traversed the globe, building an army of young people dedicated to fighting social injustice.

II. COUNTERING FAILURES OF IMAGINATION

Six weeks into the job, cholera appeared in Haiti for the first time in at least a hundred years. This nineteenth-century disease persisted throughout the twentieth and early twenty-first centuries in many settings where poverty also persisted. But somehow Haiti—long labeled the "poorest country in the Western Hemisphere"—had been spared until October 2010, nine months after a magnitude 7.0 earthquake leveled much of the capital city, Port-au-Prince. Within days of the cholera outbreak, it looked unlikely that the local and international response in Haiti would be sufficient to prevent great suffering and death. Paul immediately got to work, seeking to reverse the cruel fate that seemed to await this beleaguered country in which he's worked for three decades.

In Paul's class, we had learned how failures of imagination undermined global efforts to respond to AIDS, tuberculosis, cancer, and other modern plagues.[3] When dealing with the health problems of the poor, public health policymakers often adhere so strictly to the doctrine of "cost-effectiveness"—a valuable tool for setting priorities, but just one tool among many—that responses to the big challenges in global health are anemic. Only inexpensive medical care is deemed appropriate for settings of poverty. Paul has a pithy expression for this perverse outcome: "cheap shit for the poor." (He left that one out during class.)

When used in a vacuum, cost-effectiveness analysis at times produces incorrect and unethical claims. To cite just one example, a 2002 study concluded that in Africa it is 28 times more cost-effective to prevent new HIV infections than to treat people who already have AIDS.[4] The authors thus effectively recommended letting 25 million people—all those living with AIDS in Africa at the time—die because they thought it would be too expensive to save them. How could well-meaning people make such a monstrous (and ill-founded) suggestion? Is anyone authorized to wield instruments like cost-effectiveness analysis with such certainty when so many human lives are at stake? These are questions Paul takes up throughout this volume.

The short answer is that claims such as these are failures of imagination. The authors of the 2002 paper arrived at their conclusion by treating "cost" and "effectiveness" as givens, but both turned out to be highly variable. Consider cost. Within a decade, the cost of AIDS therapy dropped from $10,000 per patient per year to less than $100 per patient per year. Meanwhile, AIDS drugs proved more effective than initially thought. Not only do multidrug regimens suppress the virus indefinitely, they also reduce transmission by 96 percent.[5] Put simply: treatment works as prevention, too. Today more than 8 million people are on treatment worldwide; some 6 million of them live in Africa.[6] Few experts of any stripe could have imagined, in 2002, just how cost-effective AIDS treatment really is.

As this example reveals, global public health experts have sometimes become the tools of their tools, to paraphrase Thoreau.[7] This is a problem when dealing with lethal infectious diseases that cross borders and burn through the ranks of the poor. The quick fix will never be enough to contain the really difficult diseases or protect the populations most vulnerable to them.

We learned this lesson, once again, in Haiti. In late 2010, the World Health Organization and other public health heavyweights got to work making policy recommendations about cholera in Haiti. Instead of using every weapon in the arsenal, as would have happened had the disease appeared in the United States or any other wealthy country, the post-quake aid apparatus balked, opting to promote certain interventions over others. In particular, oral cholera vaccine was ruled out as "too expensive" or "too complex to deliver" in Haiti. As Paul's students know, these are precisely the arguments used to lowball the global response to malaria, drug-resistant tuberculosis, AIDS, heart disease, mental illness, and many other afflictions of the world's poor. And they are spurious arguments: the vaccine is administered orally and costs only $3.70 for the two required doses; increased production would lower prices even further. Providing health care doesn't get much easier than that. Accompanying Paul from policy meetings in New York to cholera treatment facilities in Haiti, I felt like I had a ringside seat as the latest installment in the sorry history of global health ran its course.

Predictably, the cheaper approach did not stop cholera. Within weeks, the epidemic had spread across the country, tracing a grim map of the scarce access to safe drinking water and modern sanitation across Haiti. Thousands have since perished from a disease that can in most cases be treated with simple rehydration, and transmission continues at alarming rates. The epidemic in Haiti is now the world's largest in half a century.

Could a more forceful and a truly comprehensive response— one that integrated cholera vaccine with other interventions— have stopped cholera? We'll never know, but surely it would have slowed the pace of the epidemic. It might have saved thousands of lives.

A year and a half after cholera hit Haiti, PIH finally got the green light to roll out a modest vaccination campaign in conjunction with its Haitian sister organization, the Haitian Ministry of Health, and another Haitian medical nonprofit. From April to June 2012, about 100,000 Haitians received the two-dose vaccine course in rural and urban Haiti. It is too early to claim success, but the news has been only positive to date: demand for the vaccine is high in the population, and the Ministry plans to scale up the campaign across the country with support from the United Nations and many other organizations. The World Health Organization recently endorsed the initiative, too. Long-term control of cholera will require building robust water and sanitation systems across Haiti, which will take time.[8] In the interim, it would be foolish not to use every weapon we've got to help slow the world's worst cholera epidemic in recent memory.

Failures of imagination—claiming that you can't treat AIDS in Africa or that you can't deliver cholera vaccine in Haiti—and what we can do to reverse them are, in my mind, what this book is all about.

III. ACCOMPANIMENT

Why is it acceptable to lower our standards when considering the health problems of the poor? How might we usher in a bolder chapter in the history of global health? The speeches in the first section ask readers to think hard about these questions. Paul encourages us to *reimagine* equity: what kind of world do we want to live in? What might our world look like if the next generations take poverty and inequality seriously? What kind of movement will it take to bring this vision into being?

One necessary part of a movement for global health equity is a cohort of medical professionals dedicated to serving the poor. In Paul's commencement speeches at medical schools, many of which appear in the second section, he asks new doctors to keep in mind the big picture: all that lies beyond cutting-edge laboratories and clinical facilities. The upper echelons of health research and practice in the wealthy world embody the promise of modern medicine. But without an equity plan, that promise remains unrealized to billions of people around the world—the very people who shoulder the lion's share of the burden of disease. Paul isn't calling for everyone to drop what they're doing and start working on the frontlines of global health. He's always been a stalwart cheerleader for scientific innovation, and commends all those who devote their lives to pushing the frontier. He just asks that every member of the medical professions, broadly defined, remember that even the greatest therapeutic or diagnostic breakthroughs will mean little unless they reach the people they were designed to help.

Paul also encourages new doctors to remember the importance of old-school caregiving.[9] He sums up the simple business of caring for others—visiting them in their homes, helping them fill prescriptions, washing their dishes—in a word that appears throughout this volume: accompaniment. Doctors and nurses and community health workers should, Paul suggests, be *accompagnateurs* (a word adopted from Haitian Creole) to their patients. The practice of accompaniment is one of the main reasons why PIH achieves outstanding clinical outcomes when treating complex diseases like cancer, drug-resistant tuberculosis, AIDS, and depression in some of the poorest parts of the world.[10] By attending to the social and economic deficits that deny billions of people fundamental human rights—the topic of this book's third section—PIH teams attack ill health at its root: poverty, joblessness, homelessness, hunger, decrepit schools and hospitals, a lack of municipal water and sanitation systems. As Paul reminds medical school graduates, accompaniment isn't just humane practice; it's best practice.

But, as the speeches in the fourth section make clear, accompaniment goes well beyond the clinical realm. Paul sees in it a new model for all "aid" work. What does "accompaniment" really mean? Although it might at first seem simple, I think it is among the most difficult concepts to grasp in the speeches that follow. But there might be no more important principle animating Paul's work and vision. In his own words, then:

> "Accompaniment" is an elastic term. It has a basic, everyday meaning. To accompany someone is to go somewhere with him or her, to break bread together, to be present on a journey with a beginning and an end. . . . There's an element of mystery, of openness, of trust, in accompaniment. The companion, the *accompagnateur*, says, "I'll go with you and support you on your journey wherever it leads. I'll share your fate for a while"— and by "a while," I don't mean a little while. Accompaniment is about sticking with a task until it's deemed completed—not by the *accompagnateur*, but by the person being accompanied.[11]

Accompaniment is different from aid. "Aid" connotes a short-term, one-way encounter: one person helps, and another is helped. Accompaniment seeks to abandon the temporal and directional nature of aid; it implies an open-ended commitment to another, a partnership in the deepest sense of the word.

Partners In Health was founded on the notion of accompaniment. Paul, and everyone at PIH, pledged to take this longer, more unpredictable road in serving the poor. They brought resources—medical, human, financial—but instead of imposing their own agenda on their intended beneficiaries, they formed partnerships and resolved always to accompany, not to lead. PIH sought to replace the hubris of traditional foreign assistance with humility, trust, patience, and constancy—to replace aid with accompaniment.

This is not an easy approach. It entails radical availability. (Paul rarely stops working, despite frequent attempts by friends and family to get him to take a vacation.) It means investing in ambitious projects that take years to complete and are unlikely to produce frequent bursts of measurable outcome data, as demanded by many donors concerned with impact evaluation.[12] And it means always trying again when projects fail. "It's not easy to admit, even today," Paul writes in one of the speeches in this volume. "We tried and mostly failed. . . . Haunted by mediocrity, we keep returning to the task of raising the standard of care."[13] This dogged commitment to doing whatever it takes to give the poor a fair shake is the essence of accompaniment.

. . .

Over the last two years, I've learned a little bit about what it means to be an accompagnateur. Paul is the first to say that everyone needs accompaniment, and that includes Paul, the consummate accompagnateur himself. Beneath his irrepressible good humor lie enormous cares and, as he describes in the speeches that follow, doubts and fears. Trying to be his accompagnateur isn't easy for any of us on his team. Despite regular all-nighters and feverish last-minute scrambles, it is hard to catch up to Paul's steady, burning commitment to fighting injustice. We struggle with feeling inadequate, frustrated, and trivial; sometimes we want to leave work with an evening ahead. "Radical availability" is a physical, mental, and emotional challenge. With time, however, I realized that even small steps toward a more inclusive and compassionate vision, toward accompaniment of any measure, can earn you membership in Paul's army. Probably none of us can do as much as Paul Farmer has done to bend the arc of history toward justice. But as Paul reminds us throughout this volume, no matter what paths we tread, each of us can strive in some way, however small, to be an accompagnateur to those who have not been blessed by good health and good fortune. And in so doing, we are, one baby step at a time, helping to repair the world. If my generation and the generations that follow take Paul's entreaty to heart, I have little doubt we can expand the promise of modernity—the chance at a life free from poverty and premature death and unnecessary suffering—and move the world toward equity, peace, and prosperity.

PART I

Reimagining Equity

For most of us, the phrase "modern medicine" brings to mind the rapid development of health interventions since the mid-twentieth century and the sharp declines in mortality they have brought to many parts of the world. And it should. The progress of medicine and public health in the last sixty years has been nothing short of stunning. But such cheering often obscures the fact that so many simply don't have access to health care, period. This was the take-home message, as my medical students say, of the first speech in this volume, "General Anesthesia for the (Young Doctor's) Soul."

Anesthesia is more than a metaphor here. Diminution of pain, whether during childbirth or during the course of surgical intervention, is the goal of anesthesia. Lessening suffering can be seen as a quest of modernity and even as a marker of civilization.[1]

When historian Drew Faust described the American civil war as "the late middle ages of medicine," she meant that the mechanization of war outpaced any real ability to lessen either the suffering of the injured or the infectious complications of

3

overcrowding and battlefield surgery.[2] Of the estimated 750,000 killed during this conflict, most were felled by "camp epidemics"—typhoid fever topped the list—or by staphylococcal and streptococcal complications of wounds and amputations. This was indeed the dark ages of medicine and public health.

Great progress has been made since 1865. We have seen remarkable technological advances in biomedicine; plagues that once claimed countless lives are now treatable and sometimes preventable. The difference between 1865 and the present holds in one concept: triage. The line drawn between those with a chance of survival and those given up for dead has been steadily pulled in, with more and more desperate cases becoming manageable cases.

But the fruits of modern medicine have been slow to reach those in greatest need of them: the poor and otherwise vulnerable. Poverty operates its own triage on civilian populations. The poor are saddled with the greatest share of disability and disease even as they are deemed less worthy objects of health care by a medical establishment that privileges *ability to pay* over *need*. In settings of privation, medical personnel are socialized for scarcity and failure in a way reminiscent of the practitioners of battlefield medicine in ages past. We are urged to avoid "wasting" resources on groups of people who are not expected to make significant improvement. In the face of such stinginess, doctors and nurses working in settings of poverty must resist the impoverishment of aspirations.[3]

This ratcheting down of expectations for the sick and poor takes us in the opposite direction from the proper aspiration of all global health work: a world in which the poor and sick get their fair share of our planet's vast resources, medical and otherwise. But the medical profession has too often left equity for others to worry about.[4]

We fail to think about equity because we are anesthetized. This kind of anesthesia—the bad kind—occurs chiefly because we live in a violently unequal world. In the speeches reprinted here, I've drawn a distinction between *event violence*, such as war and genocide, and the insidious *structural violence* that accompanies poverty and inequalities of all sorts. Psychological, moral, or economic anesthesia dulls us most effectively to structural violence. We interpret disparities in health and income and good fortune as "the way things are." Structural violence is never anybody's fault.

Inequalities of risk and outcome—and our toleration of them—are evidence of the effectiveness of such anesthesia.

When giving a graduation speech, one is speaking to an audience of people who have been socialized for success: graduates of top-tier American universities and their families. Most have not seen battlefields, nor have they lived in settings of impoverishment and instability, which can be found in every country. Many have, however, visited or worked briefly in such places, and some have struggled with an alienation common among young people of privilege who are beginning to understand their good fortune. Some turn away from the work of repairing the world because of the pain of this alienation; others, because of the many discomforts, not all of them psychological, that are native to social justice work. I was invaded by similar feelings and doubts during my first years in rural Haiti and experienced them again more than 25 years later, when that country, my greatest teacher, was hit by an earthquake that took a quarter of a million lives.

How to bring focus and reflection to issues of equity and anesthesia? Perhaps stories communicate best. Most of these speeches, from "General Anesthesia for the (Young Doctor's) Soul" (2001) to "Countering Failures of Imagination" (2012) turn on personal experiences, my own or others'. I haven't wanted to cause pain—to withdraw anesthesia—but to make room for awareness of some ugly facts we all know anyway, to some degree. It's my conviction that poverty and inequality are the two ranking problems facing our crowded and beautiful planet—not the only problems, but perhaps the most severe, and two that, if addressed, could bring us a little closer to tackling some of the other ones.

General Anesthesia for the (Young Doctor's) Soul?

Brown Medical School, Commencement

MAY 28, 2001

Last Monday, sitting in clinic in rural Haiti, I realized that I was sweating for two reasons. One, it was seasonably hot. We always sweat in clinic. Two, I was frightened about giving this address. The fear itself had two sources. One, it's a great privilege to be here on this day, the day of your oath taking and transformation. Two, most graduation speeches are boring and forgettable. (Some are memorable largely because they are so boring.)

This latter realization struck fear in my heart. I sat there, hearing the multitudes outside, and tried hard to think of a single scrap, a word, an idea from a commencement address heard in high school, college, medical school, or grad school. But not one of them stuck. I say this apologetically, of course, since good things must have been said. I was inattentive or perhaps engaged in overly robust celebration afterward. I'm not sure what happened, but it was neither a neurologic nor a vascular event that erased these speeches. (Nor, I must add as an infectious disease guy, was it an embolic event.) The speeches never got logged in!

7

On that Monday, I knew I had one week to find what might be called the roach-motel approach: speeches check in, but they don't check out. How could I find a way to get in your heads and stay?

On Tuesday, I did a literature search. We don't have access to MEDLINE in rural Haiti, so I went into my own library.[5] I've been living in Haiti for a long time, so let's just say I have a big, if uneven, collection. Graduation, graduation. I remembered something from the English writer P. G. Wodehouse about a memorable graduation speech. It was a story of a certain Augustus Fink-Nottle, a bookish herpetologist who's gang-pressed into delivering the commencement speech at a boys' school. I recalled that Gussie, like yours truly, was terrified and did something, I couldn't remember what, to make it memorable.

After clinic was over, I found the story. Rereading it did not inspire calm. In fact, where I'd once laughed, I now found myself sweating and trembling. Fink-Nottle, normally an abstemious chap, had gotten smashed before going on stage. Gussie proceeded to insult distinguished members of the audience and to accuse the winner of the prize for scripture knowledge of cheating after the kid failed to answer the question "Who was What's-His-Name—the chap who begat Thingummy?" Wodehouse draws conclusions about speeches: "It just shows what any member of Parliament will tell you, that if you want real oratory, the preliminary noggin is essential. Unless pie-eyed, you cannot hope to grip."[6]

This counsel did not help me grip. Getting pie-eyed in the morning would be frightening enough even when you don't have to drive from Boston to Providence. Surely there was something else I could do if I wanted to make a memorable point or two?

I scarcely slept on Tuesday night, as my nightmares included a slurred speech punctuated by insults to your dean.

On Wednesday, I decided to base my Brown intervention on data. The problem called, clearly, for more research. I mean, what sort of Harvard faculty could conclude otherwise? I conducted a double-blind, controlled study of the entire population of central Haiti. I flew in a large research team and expensive consultants from the Harvard School of Public Health.

The survey showed a statistically significant correlation between amnesia and graduation speeches. Granted, the N was small: this was central Haiti, where not many have had the privilege of going to high school, much less graduate school. But chi-square tests do not lie: the picture was grim if I followed the norms. I trembled with fear, not malarial rigors. Would I have to do what Gussie Fink-Nottle had done? Do you need a designated driver in order to deliver a good graduation speech?

On Thursday, I fasted and prayed. I lit incense. I chanted and sat in the lotus position until I had bilateral nerve palsies. The medical staff and patients wondered what on earth was wrong, since I am usually a rather reliable guy. And still no inspiration came.

On Friday, I bit the bullet and did what we do in internal medicine: I called a consult.

Deep in the Haitian hills there lives a wise woman. She's called a "mambo," which translates in Hollywood-speak to "voodoo priestess." I've known her for years, and she's said to have an answer for everything. She's a bit like the woman who bakes cookies in *The Matrix*, and especially so on that day as she was sitting on a low chair stirring something in a charred pot.

I laid out my dilemma. A pregnant pause ensued; my mambo friend did not look up from her work.

"First, why are they asking *you* to talk to them? Are they going to become tuberculosis specialists or something? Fever chasers? What?"

"No," I said, "they're a mix. You know, psychiatrists to surgeons. Scientists, too."

"Well, that's good," she said. "We need all types, as they so often say, however insincerely, in your country. But it still doesn't explain why they'd want *you* to talk to them."

This was a bit too much like that part of *The Matrix* where the cookie lady tells Neo that he's not the one. I must've looked crestfallen, since the mambo continued in a kindlier tone.

"Who else will be there?"

"The students' parents and their teachers and their deans. And other sundry kin."

"Ah yes," she added. "Their 'significant others,' as you say in your country."

"Yes. I am very nervous about it because I would like to say something meaningful but have only a few minutes."

"I see your problem," she said, still stirring, "and I'm starting to remember something. A recurrent dream. What school is this?"

"Brown," I said.

She started, looked up from her pot, and smiled broadly. I knew she'd never left Haiti, at least not in the flesh, so I was wondering what was up.

"Brown! Now I understand the meaning of my dream!"

I took this to be a good sign but was puzzled.

"Look over there, child. What do you see?" She gestured to her left without looking up. A hummingbird hovered over a bush with bright red blossoms.

"A hummingbird," I said. But the word in Creole is *wanga*

neges, which means "woman charm." It can be ground into a powder with power not to give meaningful speeches but rather to seduce women. I failed to see the relevance to my dilemma and knew that crude pre-feministic tactics are frowned upon at Brown. Besides, seduction of the entire audience was the goal.

"Yes, indeed. The wanga neges. In Latin, *archilochus colubris.* And where is it?" (This, theatrically.)

"It's buzzing over the hibiscus bush near your temple." The Creole word for hibiscus is *choublak,* which comes, it is said, from the U.S. military occupation of Haiti earlier in the last century: the blossom was used to shine the soldiers' boots. Shoe black. Pretty flower, ugly name.

"What color is its throat?" she asked.

"Red."

"No, silly, its throat is brown. This is relevant, since brown is a blend of white and black and yellow and red. Remember, too, that the heart of the woman charm beats 1,200 times per minute when feeding, faster than any other creature. Now, where is the talk to be delivered?"

"Providence, Rhode Island."

"Providence! On an island! That's really amazing. It all makes sense!"

"No, well, it's not really an island."

"You don't say? And I suppose 'providence' is happenstance, too? Unrelated to my dream?" She raised an eyebrow—archly, I thought.

"Look," I said, mustering a bit of pride, "what are you getting at?"

"Don't end sentences in propositions! It's all very clear now. You are going to the university that is brown to speak to them of providence, and to remind them that they are not really living on an island. Like the word *choublak,* which is both beautiful and ugly, you'll say something that is harsh but you will say it in a nice manner. You will fly there like a bird and not row in a boat, even though a boat is necessary to reach most islands."

"Ah," I said, "so that's what the hummingbird means?"

"No silly. The hummingbird means that you will charm them, even though your heart is beating fast."

Stunned, I said nothing. It really did seem to hold together. But how would that help me with my speech?

"Look, I will give you four suggestions," she concluded gravely, "not counting the one about prepositions. First, remember that it's permitted to be anecdotal in such instances; you should talk about your poorest patients. Second, do not quote either Dickens or Shakespeare; use no Latin. Keep it heavy but light. Third, you can't please everyone in such a diverse audience. Focus on those receiving their degrees but don't try to get cute with them. For example, don't say 'Yo, what up?' when you start. Fourth, because it's Brown, be careful to offend no one. They're very sensitive about that there, it is said. You can be PC and still get to the point."

I took careful notes, thanked her, and left with new purpose. I had an entire weekend to get ready.

Now that you've heard the story about how I pulled these remarks together, you're more than halfway there! Allow me to make one last prefatory comment before I discuss providence with a small "p" and make, as did my mambo friend, four points. I'm not one of those who thinks that one medical specialty is somehow superior to another. Sure, I joke with the cardiologists at the Brigham about how exciting their work must be diagnostically—all their patients have the same disease! And I also like the occasional joke about how best to hide something from the orthopedic surgeons: put it in the literature. But I hope to address all of you, from future pathologists to budding (sorry) endocrinologists. Allow me to salute you, in typical Brown fashion, as "differentially abled" physicians. What I'm about to say is meant to be applicable to all branches of medicine and medical research.

Providence. Good fortune, whether merited or not. You are going through the transformation even as medicine undergoes a great change. I use the word "transformation" because the moment is so often transformative: you will now be asked to worry about others, many of them perfect strangers, more than yourselves. And not just anyone: the sick and vulnerable. Of course, almost all parents—and, may I add, especially mothers—do this whenever needed. But you're not doing this because your patients are your children. You're doing it because your patients are your patients and deserve fierce loyalty and the best you can offer. That's what medicine could be about, should be about, must be about.

That part is difficult but agreed upon. (Did I just end a sentence in a preposition?) The harder questions are about who gets to become a patient. I mean *your* patient, because everyone is a patient eventually. But who has ready access to the best that medicine has to offer, much of it based on relatively recently developed technologies and all of it available—providentially, it would seem—right here? Certainly not those who need it most.

The irony, now, is the best that medicine has to offer keeps getting better—thanks in large part to the health sciences also represented here today. The big leap forward that physics made a century ago is now happening in medicine. That's good news. The bad news is that unless we make *equity* our watchword, we become party to a process that promises to reserve its finest care for those who need it least, leaving billions of sick people without decent medical care.

All four points were hidden in there. But now, as the game show host says, in question form please.

I.

To whom do we owe primary allegiance? To the sick, of course, and that's easy enough to figure out on a busy call night because they're in your face. But what if they're not in your face? What if you're busy in the lab, making medical progress possible? We all know that the burden of disease lies most heavily on the poor or otherwise marginalized and yet they do not receive the best care. So far, when physicians have banded together, we've fought mostly for ourselves. In the future, our allegiance to the sick must be stronger, even, than our allegiance to one another. Otherwise we start to slide down a slippery slope. I refer here not to the slope from Percocet to Versed to Halothane. I refer to the unintentional slide toward general anesthesia for the soul. When under such anesthesia, we can function in most settings but risk missing the great moral questions that face modern medicine. That brings me to the second question . . .

II.

Why, exactly, should we fear general anesthesia for the soul? As any intern can tell you, there's nothing wrong with some oblivion after a hard night on call. But general anesthesia for the soul threatens to cheapen medicine; indeed, it already has. We can still point with pride to the difference between a vocation and a job. Now more than ever, however, medicine needs to be about service rather than conventional rewards. Curing, preventing, easing pain and suffering, consoling—these are both our "product" and our reward.

The commodification of medicine—health services for sale—continues apace without measures for caring for those who cannot pay. Soon we risk hearing, even in casual speech, the words of Plato, who in *The Republic* asked, "But tell me, the physician of whom you were just speaking, is he a moneymaker, an earner of fees, or a healer of the sick?"[7] (Note that I am not breaking the Latin Rule, as Plato was Greek, not Roman.)

Even in this affluent country, physicians have failed to make sure that all citizens have health insurance; most physicians are not yet active participants in this debate. In much of the rest of the world, including the countries in which I work, it's much worse. Equity of access was one thing in the era of leeches but quite another in our times. And the most peculiar thing about our times, as far as medicine goes, is related to important changes in technology. This segues to the third question.

III.

What will be different about medicine in the twenty-first century, and how are these changes related to general anesthesia for the soul? The short answer: well, medicine is actually effective now. Or could be. I can't very well mumble something about the best of times and worst of times, as that would be breaking the mambo ground rules, but think about it: no matter what specialty you've chosen, your practice will be completely different from that of only a single generation ago. The human genome is sequenced. Drugs are now designed rather than discovered. Surgical procedures are safer, less invasive. Diseases deemed untreatable as recently as a decade ago are now managed effectively.

But each of these triumphant truths must be qualified by "for some." Your generation will have to deal with a growing outcome gap as some populations have ready access to increasingly effective interventions while others are left out in the cold. Worse, those excluded are those who would benefit most.

Just take AIDS, the latest rebuke to hope. Over the last five years, AIDS deaths in this country have dropped sharply. So have HIV-related admissions to our hospitals. This is due, in large part, to the development of better therapy targeting the virus itself. But these advances have served only a tiny minority of those who stand to benefit. For most living with HIV, life-saving drugs are unavailable. There are all kinds of excuses. The tools of my trade—again, I'm an infectious-disease doc—have been termed "not cost-effective" in an era in which money is worshipped so ardently that it's difficult to attack market logic without being called a fool or irresponsible. Treating AIDS in a place like rural Haiti, which lacks health infrastructure, is dismissed as "unsustainable" or not "appropriate technology."

Each of these ideas, from cost-effectiveness to sustainability, could be a means of starting conversations or ending them. But in my experience in international health, arguing that treatment is not cost-effective is largely a means of ending unwelcome conversations about the destitute sick. On page 6 of the *New York Times* of April 29, 2001, you can hear a high-ranking official within the U.S. Department of the Treasury object to a strategy that would make HIV drugs available on the continent on which they are most needed. According to the article, "He said Africans lacked a requisite 'concept of time,' implying that they would not benefit from drugs that must be administered on tight time schedules."[8] These ideas stop conversations because many who would continue them are under deep anesthesia.

This leads me to the fourth question, which is no doubt on your minds as you pick up your diplomas.

IV.

What is the key step in the Krebs cycle?[9] OK, that's a joke. Heavy yet light, she said.

The fourth question: what will be the yardstick by which we gauge our success as a profession? Answering a question about the future calls for prophetic powers, and my mambo is not here. But I believe we'll be judged by how well we do among the destitute sick. Strategies designed to prolong life into the tenth decade will flourish in the affluent world, but only if general anesthesia puts all souls to sleep will history judge us by the longevity of the affluent. No, discerning judges will look instead for falling life expectancies among the poor, wherever they live.

What will historians of the future say about our actions over the past decade, during which 10 million African children were orphaned by AIDS, a decade in which life expectancies have plummeted in Haiti and a dozen other countries? And where life expectancies do rise for the poor, what of the fact that they rise so much more slowly for some than for others?

Many have documented the impact of poverty and social inequalities on the distribution and outcomes of infectious diseases. Working in Haiti or in a slum in Peru or in a prison in Russia, these are our priorities. But what about in affluent settings? What about with noncommunicable diseases? The *New England Journal of Medicine* has published studies documenting the impact of racism in choice of strategy for the management of coronary artery disease. After learning that African Americans are less likely to be referred for cardiac catheterization than whites with the same indications, do we really think that enalapril is more effective in whites with left ventricular dysfunction than in blacks with LV dysfunction for *biological* reasons? An acute editorial accompanying this study, published in the *Journal* earlier this month, draws different conclusions:

> It is indisputable that social perceptions of what a person is or is not influence the availability, delivery, and outcome of medical care. It is incontrovertible that these perceptions apply with dismaying regularity to black people and other minorities in the United States. And it is undeniable that lifestyle, socioeconomic status, and personal beliefs are powerful influences on health. But these are matters of morality and culture, and we must clearly distinguish them from the biologic aspects of race-based medicine—from the danger of attributing a therapeutic failure to the patient's "race" instead of looking for the real reason. . . . Research to root out social injustice in medical practice needs continued support, but tax-supported trolling of databases to find racial distinctions in human biology must end.[10]

Social injustice in medical practice. Science has revolutionized medicine but there was no revolution and no plan for ensuring equal access. *Excellence without equity* is what you now inherit. It's the chief human rights problem of twenty-first-century medicine, and only when we're all under general anesthesia of the soul will we be able to ignore it as the century marches on.

So what, dear Class of 2001, do we need from you? We need excellence with equity, of course. And here's the part I'd ask you to remember. We need you to shape the profession so that there's commitment to equitable service in the face of growing inequalities of outcome; we need humility and resolve in the face of bold technological advances. Note that you can change the order around—service, humility, inequality, technology—and make that into a nice mnemonic, if you like.

And there you have my graduation speech. I hope, dear colleagues, that I have kept it heavy but light. I hope that even without a powdered hummingbird I have managed to charm. I feel lucky to be here, certainly, on the very day that you all make that marvelous transformation from students to physicians. I hope that you go out there and seize medicine with both hands, with your heads and hearts, and force science and technology to serve the sick. For science and technology will and should be the heart of modern medicine, but you must add the soul. You are, providentially, products of the finest medical education in the world. Resisting the easy anesthesia that privilege affords is going to be your next big challenge.

Thank you, congratulations, and good luck.

Epiphany, Metanoia, Praxis: Turning Road Angst into Hope—and Action

Boston College, Commencement

MAY 23, 2005

Ladies, gentlemen, fathers, sisters, parents, families, graduates: surely you don't blame me for being nervous. It's been a while since I sat in that seat, and I don't want you all to find this boring or irrelevant. A week ago, a friend emailed me an article from the *Boston Globe* about how commencement speakers are chosen. It sent a chill right through me: "The graduates almost always prefer well-known figures, particularly from the entertainment world, in hopes of a speech that will provide a lighthearted finale to their college years, college administrators say."[11] The article, which mentioned Boston College and yours truly, noted that students preferred—and vocally so—speakers like Ali G and Jon Stewart. As my mother would say: "oh, boy."

So, terminally unhip, I'm going to stick with what I know best: Haiti and Rwanda, health and human rights. For all of you who take pride in BC's cosmopolitan culture and secular success, I warn you further that I'm going to frame my remarks today around a couple of concepts I learned growing up Cath-

20

olic: epiphany, metanoia, and praxis. But don't worry—I won't talk about theology and still less about philosophy or any particular faith tradition. I'll confess right here that for years I thought "epiphany" was either a hot young starlet or a Latin American vacation day; I was pretty sure that "metanoia" was a heavy-metal band whose members trashed hotel rooms and ended up in rehab; and, for the longest time, I thought a "praxis" was a disease-transmitting insect indigenous to the part of Amazonia shared by Brazil, Peru, and Venezuela.

Epiphany, metanoia, praxis—these were, the priests assured us dazed kids, very important concepts. But you'd all be disgruntled if I wasted this important day by asking you to remember three arcane Greek words. After all, you quite reasonably want your commencement speaker to say something like, "Go forth and conquer! The world is your oyster! Give 'em hell!"

Now, granted, "give 'em hell" is not a common way to kick off a speech at a Jesuit institution, but I've cleared this with Father Leahy, who pointed out, quite gravely, that the term "hell" is perfectly acceptable in theological discourse.[12] He was less pleased, however, with the vulgar contraction "'em."

Hell. What on earth is "hell"? Today's question, more properly posed, is "What is hell on earth?"

That's what you guys need to figure out because you are setting forth, at the height of your powers, into a world in which some have so much and others have next to nothing. I've met several members of the Class of 2005 and know just how talented and committed you all are. You will—you must—find out about the world's wounds. My own guess is that poverty and power-lessness and untreated disease are hell on earth and that there's nothing God given about such conditions. They are man given. And if hell can be created by others, rather than by some inescapable force of God or nature, we humans might just have a salvific role to play.

My own authority, such as it is, draws on the fact that I'm a doctor to people who are living in the worst sort of destitution, people who would say in a flash that they are living in hell. In fact, they say this all the time. I'm talking mostly about Haiti, of course. And the man-made hell to which I refer is slavery and its after-effects. Haiti, for over a century a lucrative slave colony, became the first nation to outlaw "the peculiar institution."[13] Born of a violent slave revolt, Haiti is our oldest neighbor. We owe Haiti a lot, and we haven't always been very neighborly. More on that later.

First allow me to natter on a bit about epiphany, metanoia, and praxis. By giving a few examples, I hope to suggest how important, how life changing, these three lousy Greek words can be.

I. EPIPHANY

The term "epiphany," less obscure than the other two, has entered the popular vocabulary. I'm sure it's used in several Britney Spears ballads, and it's rumored to be the title of a forthcoming album by Fifty Cent.

To have an epiphany is to suddenly understand something that had previously escaped you. A eureka moment, like when Archimedes found that lost bar of soap in the tub, or shampoo-and-conditioner-in-one, or whatever it was he'd dropped. We've all had epiphanies—and if you're lucky you've had quite of few of them here at BC. Given the tuition, your parents have every right to be disgruntled if you've had no epiphanies at all. In such case, my advice is to fake at least one, which adds up, counting tuition and expenses, to close to a quarter million dollars per eureka.

The epiphany to which I refer concerns slavery. Not the sudden discovery by an isolated slave that slavery was evil—the slaves knew that from the get-go—but rather that of a person like you or me. Much more like you than me, though, since he was 25 years old and had just finished his schooling. This was in late eighteenth-century England at the height of the slave trade.

Like many of you, Thomas Clarkson was ambitious, bright, and ready to set out to do something good in the world. He looked forward to a career as an Anglican minister. We know a lot about Clarkson. "Over six feet tall," we read in Adam Hochschild's wonderful new book, *Bury the Chains*, "Clarkson had thick red hair and large, intense blue eyes that looked whomever he spoke to directly in the face."[14]

Like some of you here today, Clarkson submitted, prior to graduating, an original piece of scholarship, an essay about slavery (an enterprise in which England was deeply invested). "His essay," recounts Hochschild, "won first prize. Clarkson read it aloud in Latin to an audience in the university's majestic Senate House, where such ceremonies are still held today. His studies finished, already a deacon in the Church of England, he mounted the horse he owned to head for London and for what seemed a promising career."

All this was prior to proper roads, and it was prior to road rage, too. But Clarkson had, en route to London, a severe attack of *road angst*:

Riding to the capital in the black garb of the clergyman-to-be, he found himself, to his surprise, thinking neither of his prospect in the church nor of the pleasure of winning the prize. It was slavery itself that "wholly engrossed my thoughts. I became at times very seriously affected while upon the road. I stopped my horse occasionally, and dismounted and walked. I frequently tried to persuade myself in these intervals that the contents of my Essay [on slavery] could not be true. The more however I reflected upon them, or rather upon the authorities on which they were founded, the more I gave them credit." These feelings grew more intense at the midpoint of his journey, as he was riding down a long hill. . . . "Coming in sight of the Wades Mill in Hertfordshire, I sat down disconsolate on the turf by the roadside and held my horse. Here a thought came into my mind, that if the contents of the Essay were true, it was time some person should see these calamities to their end."[15]

Some person should see these calamities to their end. If there were a single moment at which the English antislavery movement became inevitable, it was that day in June 1785 when Thomas Clarkson sat down by the side of the road at Wades Mill. That moment would reverberate throughout the remaining sixty-one years of his life and beyond. For us today, it is a landmark on the long, torturous path to the modern conception of human rights.

Let's stop a minute, recap the road-angst part. Picture this scene: young dude, tall and ambitious, graduates and wins prize. Wears hip black threads. Only 25 years old. Has a cool ride (though there's nothing to suggest the horse was pimped out). Good in Latin, stumbles across topic, pulls all-nighter, gets the declensions right, and blows old school away with his oratory. Tools back to London to party. Finds self dazed, "disconsolate," sitting in front of some bloody mill, wondering why in God's name self is obsessed by essay topic. Just a damn essay! An exercise! Clarkson curses self: why not an essay on Etruscan pottery, a sonnet, even Beowulf? Why on earth did he have to choose *slavery*, about which he knew *nothing*? Meanwhile, horse is munching roadside greenery, staring at crazy white guy, grazing, waiting, staring, grazing. Said white guy, still disconsolate, goes wandering into woods. Horse concludes he's gone mad. Horse keeps grazing.

But something far better than madness was enveloping Thomas Clarkson. A light was dawning. A bell went off. A deep chord was struck. This, you see, was an epiphany.

And the best was yet to come, although you've already guessed it or read the book. Hochschild continues:

> Long months of doubt followed [Clarkson's] roadside moment of revelation. Could a lone, inexperienced young man have that "solid judgment... to undertake a task of such magnitude and importance—and with whom was I to unite?" But each time he doubted, the result was the same: "I walked frequently into the woods, that I might think on the subject in solitude, and find relief to my mind there. But there the question recurred, 'Are these things true?'—Still the answer followed as instantaneously 'They are.'—Still the result accompanied it, 'Then surely some person should interfere.'" Only gradually, it seems, did it dawn on him that he was that person.[16]

To summarize, dear graduates, Clarkson asked the simplest question: "Are these things true?" And he came up with the simplest answer. *Yes.* Surely someone should interfere with this man-made abomination, slavery?

And interfere he did. Clarkson and his friends and consociates, some of them former slaves, spent decades building up a movement, performing the hard chores of what we now call community organizing. From it we learn not that one person—Clarkson, say—can have great force in the world. That may be true, but the lesson to be gathered from abolitionists is that *broad social movements* can have great force in the world. Because Clarkson and a dozen or so others, many of them Quakers and a couple of them influential, began a vast campaign. They went from town to town, traveling tens of thousands of miles on horseback, collecting signatures for petitions, calling town meetings, researching the slave trade, gathering expert witnesses, compiling testimony.

Sound modern? It was. And imagine what these people were up against. They lived in a monarchy; almost no British subjects could vote. The United Kingdom derived huge profits from the slave trade; this was in part why it ruled the high seas. Sugar, rum, tobacco, and other tropical produce had become everyday staples in Europe and the emerging "new world" in which we live today—and most of these products were drenched in the blood, sweat, and tears of people kidnapped in Africa and sold as things.

I can't resist going back to Jesuit teachings for a second. Pedro Arrupe, in laying out the principles guiding the Society, reminded us of the primary importance of "a basic attitude of respect for all people which forbids us ever to use them as instruments for our own profit."[17] The millions of people who finally brought a halt to the slave trade went back to this first principle again and again. It was step one in building a modern social movement.

II. METANOIA

Step two, for Clarkson, was metanoia. Metanoia, a change of heart, can of course come in many circumstances. Symptoms, as Clarkson's horse could tell you, include obsessive ideation, shortness of breath, facial redness, sleep loss, and the desperate urge to change something. Tom Clarkson's epiphany on the way from Cambridge to London led to metanoia and then on to informed action, which some term "praxis."

Haiti was my own Wades Mill. Haiti taught me how to better understand places like Rwanda and—more to the point—how to understand my own country and its history. I first went to Haiti right after I tossed my mortarboard in the air: I was 22 years old and graduated from college with a vague plan to go to Haiti.

Turns out that a brief "visit" to Haiti was pretty hard to pull off. Haiti stayed with me. Trying to shake Haiti, I could identify with Tom Clarkson's road angst. I found myself asking the same simple question: yes or no—are these things true?

This metanoia was hard for me. The brutal sledgehammer of poverty and disease was striking the people we sought to serve; it was hard, even, to watch. But Haiti taught me a great lesson, the very lesson underpinning the revolution that brought down slavery there in 1804: human life and human values cannot have price tags attached to them.

I think it's safe to say that General Roméo Dallaire, who is receiving a much-deserved honorary degree here today, had this same epiphany and experience of metanoia when he found himself in charge of a too-small United Nations peacekeeping force in Rwanda in 1993.[18] Dallaire watched as Rwanda went up in flames and hundreds of thousands of people were murdered at close range with machetes and other crude tools. Talk about hell on earth. But the general couldn't get the troops he needed to intervene. One story from his memoir is worth recounting:

> As to the value of the 800,000 lives in the balance books of Washington, during those last weeks we received a shocking call from an American staffer, whose name I have long forgotten.
>
> He was engaged in some sort of planning exercise and wanted to know how many Rwandans had died, how many were refugees, and how many were internally displaced. He told me that his estimates

indicated that it would take the deaths of 85,000 Rwandans to justify the risking of the life of one American soldier. It was macabre, to say the least.[19]

A cost-effectiveness analysis, a price tag, applied to a peace-keeping effort in Africa. Macabre indeed. And how terrible it often feels, we have learned, to survive when so many others died.

III. PRAXIS

Dallaire has often said that what happened in Rwanda was made possible by the world's racism. The world's indifference to the fate of a large subset of humanity continues to haunt him. He wasn't able to stop the genocide, nor could he walk away from it. He wanted to make sure the lesson would not be forgotten. This put him on a path of incessant nagging about Rwanda and justice for those who'd died. That's what praxis means. This accounts for the honor you confer on him today.

But General Dallaire was not always honored. In fact, he was given a stern dressing-down by his superiors in the Canadian armed forces. He was to give up the "Rwanda business" or he'd be forced to leave the military. Dallaire, like Clarkson some 200 years before him, stuck to his principles, and so was given a "medical discharge" from the armed services. As a civilian he has only escalated his campaign for justice. It hasn't been easy. "My soul is in Rwanda," he once said. "It has never come back, and I'm not sure it ever will."

I promised I would not try to be an amateur theologian, but what could be more soulful than allowing yourself to be open to epiphany and metanoia and so to know the suffering of others? To have your road angst followed by action? To admit failure and to soldier on?

Still, I know what the general means about being haunted by experiences of hell on earth, which is to say, experiences in impoverished and war-torn regions of the world we share. It's easy to look at the world as it is and to lose hope. Can we live—move forward—without hope?

Whoa! As some of you might say, "Dude! I can't believe I just said that!" But even though the *Boston Globe* warns us that you want, in your speaker, "a lighthearted finale to your college years," I'm going to close by asking you for something.

Whatever it is you do, and you will do great things, try to *turn your road angst into hope and action.* Do it for us, do it for each other, and do it for the millions you'll never meet but who may well be affected by your action and inaction.

You don't have to be an archbishop, or the head of a peace-keeping force, or even a doctor laboring in some isolated back-water. You can transform road angst into hope and action as a teacher or an artist or a banker or as CEO of a company. Indeed, the world is counting on the next generation of Americans to think more like Thomas Clarkson and Roméo Dallaire. I make this claim because I know, from working in Haiti, that we have great power on the global stage. The world is your oyster.

See? I promised I'd get that in somehow. But while we're at it, I'd like to know who coined the oyster declaration because I've never been sure what it means. Perhaps it's just that oysters are delicious to many and repugnant to others; perhaps it's that oysters can give you hepatitis or a pearl or a nasty cut. Perhaps the world is more like an oyster than I thought.

Whatever it means, the world is in fact counting on you, per-haps more than ever before. Many of you feel its ever-increasing interconnectedness. Technological advances will continue to make ours a smaller planet (my second safe prophecy today).

I've recently been in Haiti and am soon off to Rwanda—but not in one of the awful ships that inspired Thomas Clarkson's indignation.

As someone who is on the road a great deal, I feel a deep admiration for his epiphany, metanoia, and praxis. Back then there were no frequent-rider miles or upgrades to a better saddle or a faster horse. What he and others did was hard work.

Above all, Clarkson and General Dallaire both learned the lesson that to do nothing is also to act. So *act affirmatively*—by making things happen, not just letting them happen. Aristotle said it best: "Action is the perfection of potential." We're counting on you to go forth now with all the potential you have stored up in you and act. Not "acting" in the sense of Ali G acting, but acting on your convictions.

You're going to have some road angst along the way. Let it invade you, change you, drive you to act. Whether you become doctors or lawyers or bankers or teachers or even theologians, make room for a movement to make this world—a world you'll shape decisively—a better place.

Three Stories, Three Paradigms, and a Critique of Social Entrepreneurship

Skoll World Forum, Oxford University

MARCH 28, 2008

A new year, early in the third millennium, dawns. New plagues—AIDS, drug-resistant tuberculosis, and hospital-acquired "superbugs" of all sorts—sweep rapidly across vast swaths of land, blurring national boundaries; old maladies that should've been history, such as smallpox, remain rooted in long-standing and increasingly unjust social and economic structures. Malaria, hookworm, and other parasites claim lives or simply drain energy from hundreds of millions; it's hard to work when you're tired and anemic or pregnant a dozen times before the age of 30. There are still rich people and poor people, but most economists agree that social inequalities, both global and local, have grown rapidly over the past three decades. The earth itself is tired and malnourished. Man-made environmental crises dry up lakes, wash topsoil into the seas and smother reefs, and—from what we can tell—spark huge storms. A billion people do not have safe drinking water. A war built on lies will cost, one Nobel laureate economist tells us, three trillion dollars.[20]

What cause have we for hope? As a doctor working in Africa

and contemplating the problems of our wounded earth, I acknowledge that the butcher's bill is high. Yet here we are, a gathering of what are termed "social entrepreneurs," and we *are* full of hope.[21] Some of that hope is tied to risk. Some of it is tied to an increasing awareness of the great world around us. There is, as is often reported by cheerleaders of commerce, vast and rapid growth in the global economy. China and India, not so long ago poor and agrarian, are already economic powerhouses, and these economies continue to grow rapidly if unevenly and fueled by coal and oil. With fifty years of peace, Europe is more prosperous than ever. In spite of trade imbalances, a recession, and imprudent wars, the United States remains rich, current exchange rates aside. (I thought buying a cup of espresso was bad in New York. I swear you can pay $20 for a cup here.) Our citizens, if famously ill informed about the world, are generous: almost half of American households responded to a tsunami in Asia, more than any other nation, and even more tried to respond to the worst hurricane ever to hit our country's Gulf coast.

This is a time of great problems, some new and some old, and a time for novel solutions. It's a time for social entrepreneurs.

When Sally and others at the Skoll Foundation called me last summer to let me know that, after a thorough work-up, diagnostic testing had proven that I was of this special breed, I was driving along a road in southeastern Rwanda.[22] I pulled over to express my thanks to the staff there and to Jeff. I shared with them my deep gratitude for the honor and the support of our work.

My puzzlement I kept to myself: what, exactly, is a social entrepreneur? I know I'm a doctor and an anthropologist, but part of me winced as I acknowledged that, yes, we live in an era in which simply seeking to provide high-quality medical care to the world's poorest is considered innovative and entrepreneurial. Thus the diagnosis comes with both honor and shame. Shouldn't we have long ago offered such services to those who need them most? Shouldn't we have designed systems to solve the health problems faced by the world's bottom billion?

I've learned a lot this week and made connections with others similarly diagnosed, and I think I get it now. Social entrepreneurship means many things, and those diagnosed do many things. But all of us carrying the diagnosis of social entrepreneur display certain symptoms that suggest not only the diagnosis but also that it may be infectious. Indeed, we may soon see a global pandemic of social entrepreneurship.

Here are some of the classic symptoms of the disease: refusal to accept the world the way it is, and the direction in which we're going. An unwillingness to say, no this can't be done. Persistence. A certain amount of righteous anger about the injustices done unto others, especially the poor and marginalized, and a willingness to fight back against unjust systems. And also hope. Blood tests I've done this week, clandestinely of course and while you slept, show that all of us have alarmingly high serum levels of hope. And while you dozed in your rooms in Oxford, I was doing MRIs of your brains, and so I know that you have, in fact, strategies to respond to the problems that bring us together. I hope you don't mind that I didn't get any consent forms signed.

I for one am not embarrassed by high serum hope levels, as long as our entrepreneurship remains grounded in solving real problems, especially the problems of those left behind or, worse, *damaged* by the unsustainable development that we have promoted over the past two centuries. And some have been far more damaged than others. Today I will seek to do two things. I wish to share with you some stories about transformations—personal, institutional, and political—that I've had the good fortune to witness recently in Rwanda, of all places. Rwanda has come back from the brink of hell and is the most social entrepreneurial country I have ever seen. Epidemiological studies suggest a pandemic of entrepreneurialism is breaking out there. Then I will close with comments about the Achilles heel of our nascent movement as social entrepreneurs. And, as an anthropologist, I promise to speak of culture, though not in the way you'd expect.

I.

Hope in Rwanda. This will surprise some of you. If there is one continent on which economic growth is slow or stalled or uneven, it's Africa. This is also the continent with the highest burden of the diseases mentioned above and, accordingly, the shortest life expectancy and the highest rates of maternal mortality. We've all heard the numbers before. There is no shortage of diagnoses and prescriptions for the ills of sub-Saharan Africa, and many are discrepant.

But many diagnoses and prescriptions are *not* discrepant. To the old question, can we break the cycle of poverty and disease? we have an answer: *Yes, we can.* Science, innovation, sound policy, and good governance, along with the needed resources, could close the gap between rich and poor, could promote genuinely sustainable development, which means development with social justice and less inequality. And this would lead, some of us believe, to a dampening of the violence that continues to afflict hundreds of millions, most of them poor.

People like Faustin, a child I met in rural Rwanda two years ago, are the chief victims of this violence, which is never really local and has almost nothing to do with *his* culture. On a Wednesday morning in March 2006, two boys, while herding cows, picked up a landmine. In Rwanda this is an increasingly rare event, as many efforts have been made to find and disarm such weapons. (Time will tell if Rwanda has been, as I believe, successful in lessening the chances that mass violence will ever occur there again.) Unfortunately, it is still too often a common event elsewhere: within the past decade, it has been estimated that there are 110 million landmines in the ground worldwide, and more than twice as many are stockpiled. Today, thirteen countries continue to manufacture anti-personnel devices, though as little as fifteen years ago that number was over 50 countries and almost 100 private companies, 47 of which were based in the United States. Of those who detonate the landmines unintentionally, 80 percent are civilians and one in five, children. About half die, virtually all the rest are injured and many of them are permanently maimed.[23]

Both of the Rwandan boys survived, and I came to know quite well the one who was injured more seriously, as he spent more time in the hospital and needed physical therapy, home visits, and social assistance. I met Faustin at ten in the morning on that Wednesday, as I was headed out of the hospital to a clinic a couple of hours away. The hospital was built and once owned by a Belgian mining company, which left Rwanda decades ago, having extracted what it came to extract. After the war and genocide in 1994, the facility fell into disuse, essentially abandoned until May of 2005, when we (Partners In Health, the Clinton Foundation, and the Rwandan Ministry of Health) rebuilt and opened it as the sole hospital serving more than 200,000 people, most of them resettled refugees, and almost all of them living in poverty.

By March 2006, we had cobbled together a medical and nursing staff consisting mostly of Rwandan professionals and a handful of expatriate volunteers. One of my colleagues, a physician from Cameroon, stopped me that morning, saying "Come quickly to the emergency room. Two children have picked up a grenade." At that moment I did not think it unlikely that someone in the region would have picked up a grenade and pulled the pin: after all, the boys live (and we practice medicine) in a region hit hard by the war and genocide. Ordnance hangs around for years. The boys said that they merely picked the thing up and threw it toward the cows they were herding; the cows took the full force of the mine, and two were killed. It was an hour or so after seeing the boys before I began to think about the object itself, what it was and where it had been manufactured—certainly not Rwanda. In the meantime, neither I nor my colleagues were thinking about anything other than trauma care, which is of course precisely what trauma victims need most. In this case it meant splinting fractures, debriding wounds, and applying dressings. We worked attentively and in near silence.

Of the two boys, one was not seriously injured. The other, Faustin, sustained multiple fractures, and many fragments had been blown into his skin. I had the privilege of splinting him, pulling the plastic fragments out of him, and preparing him for transport. Although we had just rebuilt the operating room, we did not have an orthopedic surgeon on staff, and Faustin needed to have his fractures set in the OR with what is called an external fixator.

Faustin, even in the course of interviews conducted at home after the device was placed, did not wish to speak of his experience. "What I'd most like to do," he said only a few days after surgery, "is to go to school." It turned out that he was not an orphan, after all, but that his mother, poor and bereft after the genocide, had struggled for years with mental illness and had finally placed him with another family in 2004. "My mother is not well," he told me later. "She can't take care of me, so she brought me to a relative and I live here now. I would like to go to school, but [my adoptive family] has no money. So I herd cows every day, make sure they eat, move them to new grass." When I asked him about the landmine, he was, astonishingly to me, apologetic: "I didn't mean to pick up the grenade. I'm sorry I did it. I didn't mean to kill the cows. I'm sorry. It was an accident. We didn't know what we were doing; it was not our intention to kill the cows."[24]

To me, as grotesque as it is to hear a child apologize for a landmine built in God-knows-what country, this is a story of hope, for the desire to go to school is as hopeful as it is universal. Faustin is now in school.

Every day we meet people who are much sicker than Faustin, but they too have some hope, or they would not have come to see us. Sometimes of course they are almost without hope, and sometimes we go to see them. Consider one of my patients named John, who had at the same time three of this century's worst diseases: TB, AIDS, and poverty. We cured his TB with antibiotics, of course, but he also received the only known treatment for hunger: something called food. Can you believe that we have to spend an endless amount of time arguing that food is the proper treatment for malnutrition? With our peers and friends? Yet we do. A few months later, John was transformed. He and I joked that he changed from looking like Skeletor to looking like someone who needed Lipitor.[25] I ran into him in the hospital last week and he reminded me that what he most wanted was a cow. Again, John has hope because he feels well enough to work; it's what he wants to do.

These are individual stories, which are not to be discounted, and I will not apologize for sharing them with you. But social entrepreneurs and our supporters are all obsessed, it would seem, with something called *scale*. The fetishization of scaling up our work is a source of both anxiety and hope. Bringing a new, innovative project to scale often feels like the only way to leave a footprint (of the good kind) in an afflicted world in need of new ideas. We have worked with the Rwandan government to scale up comprehensive care in three of the four districts in which there were no district hospitals. And, if I may brag, our Haitian colleagues have been with us from the very beginning in Rwanda. Our biggest obstacle is funding the scale-up and, again grotesquely, the battle royal over paying community health workers. There's no real argument about paying ourselves and our peers; we all get paid for our labor. It's the poor who are being asked to volunteer, and since we know that doesn't work, we are searching high and low for the modest funds to pay them. The Skoll award will go a long way in helping us to see this model adopted much more widely.

Partners In Health is now working in nine countries; we have trained and stipended thousands of community health workers serving millions. I can't imagine anything more cost-effective than that. We have established formal training programs in global health equity at Harvard and one of its affiliated teaching hospitals. These were, to our knowledge, the first such training programs, but there will be plenty more because we're living in a time in which entrepreneurship and new ideas are not only needed but valued. Global health is now almost a fad in most American universities, and I for one hope it's not a passing trend.

II.

Medicine and public health will not solve the world's problems but can offer part of the solution to some of them. What's been shocking to me over the past 25 years is the lightning speed at which many policymakers, themselves shielded from the risks faced by Faustin or John, decide that a complex intervention is "too difficult" or "not cost-effective" in Haiti or Africa, or "not sustainable." In microfinance parlance, many of my patients are "poor credit risks." But aren't they the very people we claim to serve in the first place? And this is why I wrote this speech, in part as a critique of our movement: we need to be aware that each of the terms and concepts and tools we've developed can be used to deny the destitute access to goods and services that should be rights, not commodities. They're not full participants in the magic market, after all. How many times have you heard that people will value something more if they pay for it? And yet how many times have you seen data showing this is so regarding vaccines, bednets, or external fixators after picking up a landmine? Does anyone really believe that a mother loves her newborn more if she's had to pay some sort of user fee to access prenatal and obstetric care?

Such claims are piffle, of course, but they are also deeply reflective of an ideology that has crept into the social entrepreneur movement. Indeed, this may be the Achilles heel of the social entrepreneur movement. And so—surprise—the culture I wish to speak about is our own: the culture of social entrepreneurs. Among some entrepreneurs, I've found, it's not popular to talk of rights. We speak, instead, of "product" and "brand." Patients and students—children!—become "clients" or even "customers." The notion of sustainability becomes a blunt instrument used *against* the poor. I've seen it time and time again and bet that others here have, too.

This way of seeing the world has deep roots, and one's own culture is always hard to see. It envelops us. But it is our culture we create and need to shape. To do so we need to be aware of the limitations of any culture that sees all services as commodities and very few as rights.

Let me be clear: this is not some sort of "anti-market" stance. It's merely the argument that market alone will not solve the greatest problems of our time. It's the argument that even though we're not from the public sector, we need to do everything in our power to make sure that the public sector does not shrivel and die. Why? Not only because a functioning public-sector health or education system is often the only way to bring a novel program to scale. Not only because we need the participation of governments to address the current environmental crises at the transnational scale needed to make a difference. There is another reason to fight the gutting of the public sector: only governments confer rights. The right to health care and the right to education can be moved forward by people like us, but NGOs, universities, foundations, and forward-thinking businesses are not, alas, in the business of conferring rights. And without basic rights—to water, security, health care, and the freedom from starvation—then the world's poor do not have much hope of a bright future.

Look around this famous room and you will see a conspicuous absence of poor people. You'll see people of every hue and background, but not the poor. My comment is not a rebuke: what matters is less that we invite them to Oxford and more that we fight for their right to survive and to become themselves social entrepreneurs. Without them, the movements we seek to build, and the entrepreneurship we seek to foster, will not succeed. If a movement can have two Achilles heels—and I know I've mangled the metaphor—this is the second one. We cannot build an environmental movement or a movement for sustainable development that does not have the social and economic rights of the poor at its center. And they are decidedly not there yet. The environmental movement, for example, has for too long been a movement of the privileged.

How can we help build such movements? In our culture of entrepreneurs, there are three complementary paradigms that we can draw on. I've already spoken about the human rights paradigm. The notion of a right to health care and clean water and education is largely an Enlightenment idea, but one that retains great potency. The funny thing is that, among self-proclaimed human rights experts, social and economic rights tend to be the neglected stepchildren. Last night, President Carter said as much: when he began working in rural Africa, he heard less about civil and political rights and more about the right to water, food, and health care. We've had just the same experience. The focus in what we call "the West" is largely on civil and political rights. We should not give up on the rights paradigm but rather enlarge it to include the rights of the poor. Water. Food. Health care. Jobs. Education.

There is also the public-goods-for-public-health paradigm. This paradigm is more timid but very useful among the powerful who are frightened or embarrassed by all this talk of rights. Let me give an example. When effective treatment for tuberculosis was developed, it would have been a good idea to make it available to anyone with tuberculosis, regardless of social station. To *sell* treatment for an airborne disease was not smart: those who could pay might get better, but those who could not pay would buy what they could and then develop drug-resistant TB. All this came to pass in the decade after the Second World War, and so public health experts, uncomfortable with the notion of a right to health care, began speaking of "public goods for public health." Airborne diseases are pretty clearly public problems, not private ones. A hard-won lesson.

Then, in the 1980s, came a change in culture. Instead of "health for all," we got "structural adjustment" and neoliberalism, peddled by the international financial institutions. Controlling cost, not expanding care, became paramount; discussions of rights and public health were replaced by sermons about the free market. Still one scarcely hears admission that it is wrong, in settings of great squalor, to insist on "user fees" or "cost recovery" from the poorest. This may seem a strange debate to have in Britain, but even in the United States, where I once lived in a trailer park, there was never any doubt that I would go to public school as a right, not a commodity. It didn't matter that my mother was a grocery store cashier with six children. It never occurred to me that I might not go to school or even to university. Granted, I never dreamed I'd end up at Harvard, much less become a professor there. But I knew I'd go to school, even though I knew nothing at all about taxes or the public sector.

This leads me to the third paradigm: the development paradigm. I've spoken already of the perversion of the notion of "sustainability"—anything can be sustained for us, but almost nothing can be sustained for them. Example: pay a Harvard professor a big consulting fee to work on community health care in rural

Africa but refuse to pay the village health workers as "unsustainable." This we must reject outright.

But there is a bigger argument to be made: economic development cannot occur without investments in public-sector health and education systems. A woman who will have, on average, eight pregnancies, no education, and malaria three times a year must not be expected to contribute to development. She, as often as not, will not survive to my age, which is 48. We need to link our notions of sustainable development with pragmatic efforts to safeguard the social and economic rights of the most vulnerable inhabitants of our planet.

That begins by partnering with leaders of goodwill in the public sector. Everywhere we hear stories of corrupt officials in Africa and other poor parts of the world. But I've found that such claims are exaggerated, a product perhaps of our own culture of social entrepreneurs. I have met so many leaders of goodwill in Rwanda, the nation of hope of which I spoke earlier. It is a well-managed nation, for all its tragedies and great poverty. Most of the countries with the lowest life expectancies at birth are poor. Some are mismanaged, as are some of the wealthy countries, including one I won't mention by name but know well having been born there. Still, many of the poorest countries are led by officials seeking to promote development. Social entrepreneurs need to help them respectfully without undermining the public sector. It took me over 10 years to learn this, I'm ashamed to say.

III.

Let me close by reflecting on how social entrepreneurs can be part of a genuine, broad-based social movement. I believe that when we look back over the next quarter of a century, we'll be consoled most by our contributions to a movement that continues to grow not only in villages, slums, and squatter settlements but also on campuses such as this one. It's a movement that will come to include a growing concern with the way in which the earth itself has been damaged, polluted by greed and war and feckless policies handed down from on high. But it's a movement that pays heed not only to the environment but also to the poor who are the chief victims of greed, war, and unjust policies.

Bertolt Brecht, who is almost always right, has argued that "the compassion of the oppressed for the oppressed is indispensable. It is the world's one hope."[26] I fear that, at this late date, an additional kind of solidarity is necessary. A social justice movement that links the rich world and the poor world, the Sheldonian Theater to the village in Rwanda to which I return tomorrow. A movement that links concern for the earth with respectful solidarity with its poorest inhabitants is our great hope for a world marked by less suffering and violence and premature death. It's our great hope for the generations to come, and for our own children, privileged though they may be.

We may be leaders of this movement but must also be humble participants. It's a fluid, chaotic movement, just now coalescing, but with the promise of lessening the hurts and insults of an unequal world. And it demands a little more militancy. I close by citing a new book by Paul Hawken, *Blessed Unrest*:

> It is time for all that is harmful to leave. One million escorts are here to transform the nightmares of empire and the disgrace of war on people and on place. We are the transgressors and we are the forgivers. "We" means all of us, everyone. There can be no green movement unless there is also a black, brown, and copper movement. What is most harmful resides within us, the accumulated

wounds of the past, the sorrow, shame, deceit, and ignominy shared by every culture, passed down to every person, as surely as DNA, a history of violence and greed. There is no question that the environmental movement is critical to our survival. Our house is literally burning, and it is only logical that environmentalists expect the social justice movement to get on the environmental bus. But it is the other way around; the only way we are going to put out the fire is to get on the social justice bus and heal our wounds, because in the end, there is only one bus.[27]

Sometimes entrepreneurs need to learn to be quiet passengers on this bus. Sometimes we'll take our turn at the wheel. Sometimes we'll be the mechanic. But all of us need to get on the social justice bus. That's the bus on which the real sustainable, green movement will be traveling. It's on that bus that we'll have epidemics of social entrepreneurship. Don't get on the chartered plane.

As a friend of mine likes to say, "Hope is not a plan." But we need hope and courage and a plan to end, for example, an unjust war. We need hope and energy to tackle the diseases that should have been wiped out decades ago or never allowed to spread so rapidly. We need hope to counter policies that have weakened public-sector institutions without delivering on the promise to lift all boats. We need hope to speak to people in powerful positions whose hearts, unlike the polar icecaps, show few signs of melting. We need hope and we need each other.

To Jeff and Sally and all of you who share this diagnosis with me, thank you for including me in your ranks. I'll see you on the bus.

The Story of the Inhaler

College of the Holy Cross, Commencement

MAY 25, 2012

Thank you for inviting me back to Holy Cross. I was last here as a guest of Father McFarland's in 2005, and it's an honor to share this podium with him and to be with you and your families today.[28] A lot has changed for many of us: we've been through everything from retirements to commencements, from earthquakes to reconstruction. But Holy Cross looks much as it did eight years ago. And as you, Class of 2012, head out into the world beyond, you'll find comfort in the constancy of Holy Cross and in its capacity to adjust to change, too. Change often bruises the heart but it's inevitable and necessary if you're to live up to the Ignatian ideal of "in this sign you shall conquer."

Wait—wrong motto. I meant "men and women for others."[29]

My experience as a medical professor has allowed me to meet several Holy Cross grads. One of them, Jon Niconchuk, Class of 2009, addressed your class at your freshman convocation. He's as good an example as anyone of trying to live for others—especially those who've been left behind by poverty and illness, two scourges that will figure in my remarks today.

I promise to keep this short. First, I'll tell a true story, and then I'll make three brief points.

This is the Story of the Inhaler.

In my pocket, underneath the Hogwarts get-up, is an inhaler. Even if you're not asthmatic yourself, you know someone who is. And you can imagine what it feels like to be unable to breathe, a universally distressing symptom. In this country alone, there are an estimated 25 million asthmatics, many of them children. Turns out that, among poorer kids in this country, especially in big cities, asthma remains a killer even though we have good means of preventing and treating it. So, although the Story of the Inhaler takes place in Haiti, the lessons I draw are relevant to this country and to the rest of the world. These lessons are not just for those of you heading to medical or nursing school: this is a story about unequal access to the fruits of modern science. This is everybody's problem, whether we contemplate pandemic disease or global warming. But it is, especially, *your* challenge: how we choose to build systems to deliver the fruits of science and technology is critical to our planet's flourishing in the coming decades, the very years in which you graduates become its stewards.

One day, about 25 years ago, I was in rural, central Haiti. I'd just finished my medical studies and a doctorate in anthropology. How I ended up in Haiti is part of the Story of the Inhaler. It was a college class at Duke University over three decades ago that got me interested in health disparities and in Haiti. During a research project in an emergency room, my professors helped me understand how race and class and gender (and other forces well beyond the patients' control) shaped the experiences of people in the ER and also determined who received care there for non-urgent problems in the first place.

In the Duke emergency department I met a couple of Haitians. Migrant farmworkers in North Carolina. I don't recall what brought them to the ER in the wee hours of that night, but I did get a pretty good sense of what had brought them to the United States: poverty and political repression, which often go hand and hand. I learned, too, that they didn't have access to primary care. Neither in Haiti nor in eastern North Carolina—where they harvested tobacco, sweet potatoes, bell peppers, and other produce—were they in regular contact with modern medicine. That experience piqued my curiosity about Haiti, and I went there shortly after graduating.

Within a month, I got involved in a project to introduce primary care to people who'd been displaced by the reservoir formed by Haiti's largest hydroelectric dam. My Haitian colleagues built a small clinic. It was the first modern clinic in the region, and unlike most health facilities in Haiti, the care was free (thanks to the determination of its founders and supporters). As barriers—geographic and financial—separating people from medical attention fell, we had more patients than we knew what to do with.

Although I'd been spared medical problems in my own childhood, I was diagnosed in 1984 with asthma. It was easy for me, then a student at Harvard Medical School, to get the medication I needed. It wasn't a trivial problem, perhaps, but neither was it one of my top concerns while shuttling between Haiti and Harvard. Four years later, however, I had a more serious need of medical attention. Inattentive while crossing a busy street in Cambridge, I was struck by a car. (My advice to the graduates: look both ways before crossing the street.) Lying on the pavement, I could tell my left leg was broken. After being transferred from one Harvard hospital to another, I had surgery, including a bone graft. Again, being a Harvard medical student meant I was in luck despite my bad fortune. My surgeon was the same one who attended to the New England Patriots, and I recovered promptly (although I never became a linebacker).

Since my college days, I'd tried to imagine what it would be like to be poor and sick or poor and injured. Every time I returned to rural Haiti, the reality was right in my face. In our crowded clinic, we attended to the sick and injured as best we could. We could see that much more *preventive* care was needed, and to this end we trained and salaried community health workers in dozens of villages. Part of my job back then was to visit them and their neighbors, and the Story of the Inhaler concerns one such visit made after I was able to walk again.

Though no linebacker, I loved walking, especially after my stretch of immobility. One day I walked eight miles across the dam to a village on the far side of the reservoir. The community health workers in the settlement of Wòch Milat had organized a town meeting in a thatch-roofed, dirt-floored church. They didn't have a lot of visitors down Wòch Milat way, so I got a proper welcome and was expected to say something in front of a couple hundred people. I recall talking about the importance of prenatal care, safe motherhood, and family planning.

Afterward, anxious to get back, I looked up at the gathering storm clouds. My leg was hurting by then. It was afternoon already, and getting back across the reservoir would mean a lot more walking even if we took a dug-out canoe halfway. One of Wòch Milat's community health workers asked me to see a patient. "He can't breathe," she said. I had an image, in my mind, of an older person, short of breath. I was pretty firm in my response: "No, the patient's home is not even in the same direction we're heading and it will soon be dark. If he's having diffi-

culty breathing, we need to get him to the hospital for a chest
X-ray and lab tests." I added, perhaps guiltily, "I didn't even
bring my stethoscope." I was also thinking how nice it would be
to get home to a whopping dose of ibuprofen and a glass of ice
water.

The health worker asked if I would explain that to the sick
man's wife, and I said sure. A woman who looked about 20 years
old began talking. "Yes," she replied, her husband was about her
age. "He can't breathe. Please come and see him. He's been sick
since yesterday." Frustrated, I acceded, complaining en route
that whatever he had would be better treated in the hospital after
a proper workup.

It took 45 minutes to reach the house, halfway up a mountain
and in the wrong direction. The sun was westering as we were
ushered into a tiny shack. Three children, two of them toddlers,
stood there quietly. And there, leaning against a dirty pillow
and a pile of clothes stacked on a mat on the floor, was the very
young man who, as they said, could not breathe. His name was
Jean, and his every muscle looked corded and tensed; his lips
were the color of bruises; he couldn't speak at all and looked well
past panic. From across the room, even without a stethoscope,
I could see that he was about to die of nothing other than an
asthma attack. I'd seen *status asthmaticus* several times, but only
in an emergency room, where the option of mechanical ventilation made it possible to get medications into even the stiffest
airways. "Jesus!" I said, crossing the room. "*How* long has he been
like this?"

Since yesterday, his wife responded. I couldn't imagine that
anyone could really survive a full day of this struggle. Jean did
not look like he was going to last much longer. The panic he
should have been showing suddenly flared up in my own chest.

As regards medications, I thought I'd been telling the truth when I protested I had none on me. But I did have one. Just one. I had an inhaler full of albuterol: one of the few things that might save Jean's life in this out-of-the-way outpost of Wòch Milat. But how to get the medication in him? It's not as if he could exhale, take a deep breath, and then hold it. I asked one of the community health workers to pinch Jean's nose shut—which alarmed everyone except the patient, by then too weak to struggle—while I pushed the canister into the blue plastic tube, triggering tiny doses of albuterol into the air around his mouth. I pushed again and again, trying to force some of the mist into his open mouth and down into seized-up airways. Would it work? Was it too late?

It worked. Within minutes—suspenseful, painful minutes— enough albuterol had gotten into his lungs to turn his shallow gasps into quiet wheezing. Before long, Jean sounded like a bellows. A big improvement. Jean seemed able to look at me for the first time; his rigid body went slightly slack. He was still fighting for every breath, but now could actually cooperate as we tried to get a proper dose of bronchodilator into him. Within half an hour he could even speak haltingly. "Thank. You. Doctor," he said, giving my hand a weak squeeze.

The man's wife and oldest child, a girl of about six or so, were in tears. "Thank you, thank you, thank you," they said.

A little crowd had gathered outside. Huge mounds of praise were heaped upon me. "I can't believe you were able to save him! You are a great doctor! You knew what to do immediately! You saved him!"

If I could've looked slyly at the community health workers, I might have. But my colleagues were as effusive as the patient's wife. And as Jean became slowly able to get out a few words, the young man joined right in. "You saved my life."

Technically, it was true. That is, the inhaler had saved his life. It was the only medication on my person and one used only for the treatment of acute asthma. There was no other illness I might have palliated on that afternoon, and yet that was precisely the disease poised to snuff out his young life in slow motion, right in front of his family. Since I had the inhaler in my pocket and managed to get half a dose into his lungs, I guess I *had*, technically, saved him. In any case, it was a miraculously happy moment.

It also seemed unnecessary to explain, right then and there, that it was pure dumb luck that had caused me to show up with the very drug that might make him breathe, or that I'd originally been unwilling to come to his house. I changed the subject to the prevention of similar episodes in the future, leaving the inhaler with him and explaining that we had other medicines at the clinic that would reduce the risk of another such attack. There was no point in explaining the gravity of the illness. No one on the planet understood that better than Jean.

I finally set off, in the company of my colleagues and with a trail of children and others who'd heard the story. After a ride in a small boat and then a jeep my coworkers sent for me, I was home in time for supper. A replacement inhaler was sent immediately. The ibuprofen worked its magic. I was feeling good.

And I was still feeling good the next day, when Jean came to see me. He looked completely fit and had, indeed, walked eight miles or so to get there. "I don't have words that can express how grateful I am, nor do I have worthy gifts. But I've brought you a rooster and some eggs." The praise was flowery: I had saved him; he was a second Lazarus; he would pray for me every day.

I'd heard this sort of thing many times in the preceding years and was always grateful for it but embarrassed in this instance because of the *random* nature of this save, to use your genera-tion's term. "It was an accident," I wanted to say, "not a miracle." But that too seemed to trivialize what had happened. And so I just said thank you and, after examining him and noting he was still wheezing, gave him a new set of inhalers and explained once more how to prevent future attacks or to cut them short if they recurred. "Which they will," I added. "Asthma is a chronic disease."

Less than a week later Jean was back in clinic, this time with clear lungs, a small goat, and another heaping of thanks and praise. My discomfort mounted. "It was only dumb luck," I said, coming clean at last. "Nonsense!" he replied. The half dozen or so people in earshot—in Haiti, there's always a peanut gallery—were clearly siding with Jean. "So what if you have asthma, Dr. Paul, and were walking with the inhaler for your own use? It was meant to be: you were meant to save Jean. It's clearly miraculous! Get a grip!"

To this day, more than two decades later, Jean and his family and the community health workers probably feel more or less that same way—I'd lay money on it. But it's my job, here today, to underline what the inhaler story really means in a larger world riven by inequality.

Here are my three points.

First, and most obviously: *we inhabit a bizarrely unequal planet.* This has long been true, of course. It was true in 1492, when Columbus crossed the ocean only to shipwreck off the coast of northern Haiti. It was true when Haiti became a French slave colony. It was true during the U.S. military occupation of Haiti, which lasted from 1915 to 1934. It was true more than 25 years ago when a Harvard Medical student was led unwillingly to Jean, dying on his mat.

But it's even more true today because global and local inequalities seem irreversibly to grow rather than shrink. Consider this country: thirty years ago, the much-discussed "1 percent" owned 9 percent of all personal wealth; today they claim a quarter of it. Last year, 93 percent of all new wealth generated in the U.S. economy went to the 1 percent.[30] When you move to a global scale, the numbers are even more striking: 0.5 percent of the global population holds well over a third of the world's wealth.[31] Meanwhile, some 2 billion people live on less than $2 a day. With the exception of China and a handful of other nations, most "developing countries" were poor thirty years ago and remain poor today.

The steeper the slope of inequality, the greater our challenges. This was true, apparently, in ancient Greece, when Plutarch noted that "an imbalance between rich and poor is the oldest and most fatal ailment of all republics." Such imbalances are even less tolerable in modern times. What does it mean to die unattended of a severe asthma attack in the age of Facebook or LinkedIn? If we're so linked in, what does that mean for the good stuff, such as albuterol?

Do we really lack mechanisms to share the benefits of modernity with all of our planet's inhabitants? John Maynard Keynes once argued that human society had achieved sufficient productive power to eliminate basic wants around the globe; it just lacked institutions to deliver services to those who needed them. That was in 1930.[32] Today, global productivity dwarfs that of Keynes' day, but poverty persists, and in some places deepens. I hope all of you will keep tabs on our world's growing inequalities and seek new ways of narrowing them.

Second, I've come to understand that there *is* something miraculous in the Story of the Inhaler. As much for me as for

Jean. I don't mean miraculous in some fatalistic sense, but rather *the miracle of human solidarity*, which, when linked to both meaningful action and compassion, is something all of us, all of you, can foster in your lives and work and social networks. I say "social networks" not to sound hip, but in reference to something that predated the Internet: the need, occasionally, for other people to spin us around and yank us out of our stubborn ways. The insistence of the community health workers in Wòch Milat that I turn my no into a yes was a piece of social networking, and a miraculous gift to *me*.

In the largest sense, the social network is the social safety net. Being fortunate enough to exist in webs of friendship and shared purpose requires us to be responsive, to give and to get attention, to respond not just to events but to others' evaluation of those events. If I had been acting as an isolated particle, I might have simply said no and gone home. But I was ashamed to break from my social network. This meant rethinking my no, changing it to a yes, and climbing up that hill.

Third point, and hardest one to make: *inequality and injustice can make fools of us all*. Could I really take credit for saving Jean's life? Only a fool in my shoes would mistake happenstance for destiny, or forget that only a privileged person is likely to recover from a limb-threatening injury to walk again for miles and miles. Only a person with means would end up at Harvard or Holy Cross, as student or speaker, even if we often forget that we're privileged, and that privilege comes with obligations to others and especially to the poor. Realize your good fortune, and share it with others by putting your gifts and training in the service of those who may not have had the same opportunities but are certainly appreciative of your powers to do good.

Your school, a Jesuit institution, was founded on Catholic

social teaching that reminds us of this obligation, unshirkable and imperious and beautiful. These obligations can be met in different ways today than they could when I listened to another commencement speaker drone on. But whether you work from Facebook or Twitter or YouTube, or engage in direct service, there's always room for Ignatius's reminder that we should live for others.

Let me close by quoting the talk that Jon Niconchuk delivered to your class four years ago. "I did not find myself by looking in a mirror," he said. "I began to find myself by looking out a window. Holy Cross gives you that window."

Today, you graduates stand at the window. Outside, a world of peril and promise.

Throw open that window.

Countering Failures
of Imagination

Northwestern University, Commencement

JUNE 21, 2012

I'm so grateful to share this stage with Martha Minow and the other honorees whose talents collectively lead us from evil, keep airplanes in the sky, and teach us exactly how one thing is not like another.[33] They are reason enough to be glad to be in this stadium. But then there's you: the new doctors, lawyers, engineers, teachers, journalists, and, last but not least, college graduates. It's a glorious day to be here with you.

Now, enough of this fluff. It seems unfair to me that I have to make an impression on you on this of all days. As you graduate. Not unfair in the sense of the global lottery—who is born where—but in a much more crass sense. Why is it that I must upstage last year's speaker, one Stephen Colbert? He who received hearty laughs by drawing on his well-known talent for humor, useful in such settings and about as fair as if I were to perform, right now, a minor surgical procedure on Morty Schapiro.[34] Colbert also drew on arcane knowledge of Northwestern. For example: his reference to "the rock," not a professional wrestler from Samoa but some sort of creepy hippie ritual, or his big build-up to a joke about "Dillo day."[35] Whatever *that* is. The crowd roared. Not fair, and also silly.

Let me lead with a message that I believe is of great importance for you graduates: with rare exceptions, all of your most important achievements on this planet will come from *working with others*—or, in a word, partnership.

The story I'll tell today, about a hospital in central Haiti, is a case in point. It's a story about partnerships—seen and unseen—and the power of those partnerships to bridge what seem like different worlds. Sometimes these links are forgotten. Take the Haiti-Chicago connection: some of you know that Chicago is said to have been "founded" by a Haitian. Jean Baptiste Point du Sable built a farm at the mouth of the Chicago River sometime in the late eighteenth century, making him the first non-native settler in the area now recognized as the city. Though the details of Point du Sable's early life remain a subject of debate among historians—some claim he was born on a pirate ship—it seems likely that he hailed from Haiti, perhaps even from Saint-Marc, one of the towns in the Artibonite Department where I've worked for years.

But the connections between this city and Haiti run deeper still, as the rest of this story will reveal.

I.

Travel back with me to the early 1980s, when I first went to Haiti. A college class at Duke University got me interested in health disparities and also piqued my curiosity about Haiti, where I headed shortly after graduating. I ended up in a sleepy market town in central Haiti called Mirebalais, living in the rectory of an Episcopal Church and working in a hot, overcrowded clinic.

Although not yet in medical school, it didn't take an MD to see that excellent medical care was not likely to result from a five-minute exchange with a harried Haitian doctor with no lab or other diagnostics. And it didn't require a degree in pharmacology to imagine that not many of the various potions poured into corncob-stoppered bottles there were likely to have more than a placebo effect, if that.

My job was to take vital signs and to give moral support to the beleaguered young physician. We became good friends, and in time he confessed how tired he was of working in such a shabby facility. But he never did much to change it. The doctor, not yet thirty, had been *schooled for scarcity and failure,* even as I'd been schooled for plenty and success. Even though he himself was not poor, working in that clinic had lowered his expectations about what was possible when it came to providing health care to those living in poverty.

And who could blame him? The same verdict was being drawn by most "experts" in international health at that time. As today, Haiti was the poorest country in the hemisphere and thus had one of the greatest burdens of disease; the magnitude of its challenges was difficult for me to comprehend. But the assumption that the only health care possible in rural Haiti was poor-quality health care—that was a *failure of imagination.*

I've since learned that the great majority of global public health experts and others who seek to attack poverty are hostages to similar failures of imagination. I'm one of the bunch too, of course, and am telling you this today, as you graduate, because it's taken me a long time to understand how costly such failures are. Every day in clinic offered vivid reminders of the toll exacted by a lack of imagination. It wasn't a failure to work long hours—we all did that—but rather a failure to imagine an alternative to the kinds of programs that the public health literature deemed "realistic," "sustainable," and "cost-effective"—three terms already in circulation by the late 1980s. Most of my Haitian colleagues were, like the doctor, unconvinced that excellence was possible. My experiences in Mirebalais that first brutal and instructive year inspired a lifelong desire to see, in Haiti, a hospital worthy of its people.

Mirebalais, in 1983, was also where I met Ophelia Dahl, a seventeen-year-old British student on a gap year working in an ophthalmology clinic, and also Father Fritz and Yolande Lafontant, who took me in as a volunteer. All of us had figured out, with hope and angst and revulsion, that rural Haitians deserved better medical care, and a couple years later, this group founded Partners In Health along with a few others picked up along the way. Today our organization operates a dozen hospitals and clinics across Haiti.

That was the aim: to work with Haitian partners in building the kind of health care that country deserved. It's not easy to admit, even today: we tried and mostly failed. Sometimes we succeeded: a child with acute malaria who received chloroquine; a teenager whose fractured bone was set with competence and compassion; a young woman with bacterial meningitis called back from the dead; an anemic woman in labor who was accompanied through the difficult hours of what should always be a joyous process. To be honest, when we look back at our first years of hard work and eighteen-hour days, we can't claim to have done a good job delivering quality health services. We were delivering something as hard and fast as we could. But surely the quality of the deliverables matters more than the good intentions of the caregivers or the pace of their work. The doctors graduating today will know just what I mean.

Haunted by mediocrity, we keep returning to the task of raising the standard of care. But pile on as many idealistic docs and
nurses as you like: good medical care can't be readily delivered
in low-quality hospitals and clinics. It took years and an openness to partnership, never as easy as it sounds, to build a better hospital in a squatter community—an hour up the mountain
road from Mirebalais. As we improved our services, however
slowly, the quality of the country's public facilities was declin-
ing. This was frustrating. The number of mission groups and
NGOs like ours grew, but it didn't do much for the Haitian
health system. A suspicion took hold of us that our being outside
of and unaccountable to the public sector—for all the conve-
nience that entailed—was part of the problem. We weren't adding up to the sum of our parts. We understood this more than a
decade ago and resolved to expand our work in the public sector.

II.

The decade preceding the 2010 earthquake was a time of rapid
growth for our partnership, which reached from Chicagoland
to Haiti, and there, from the Dominican border to the western
coast at Saint-Marc. But this wasn't enough to keep up with the
need.

None of us imagined that a greater affront to Haiti would
occur on January 12, 2010, at 4:53 in the afternoon, when a massive earthquake laid waste to Port-au-Prince, killing perhaps a
quarter of a million people and leaving another 1.3 million homeless. The quake forced us into the role of a disaster relief organization in addition to that of a health care provider. It also made
us completely rethink our plans to build a hospital in Mirebalais.
With Haiti's national nursing school destroyed and its medical

school damaged and closed, with most of Port-au-Prince's hospitals down or in shambles, where would the next generation of Haitian health professionals train?

Partners In Health supporters had sent thousands of donations for rebuilding. But they wouldn't be enough to rebuild something really bold and beautiful; we needed something bigger, many times bigger. The stars seemed aligned in other ways, too. One of my former students, David Walton, committed himself to a thorough overhaul and expansion of the project. His congresswoman, Jan Schakowsky, connected us to her friend Marjorie Benton, one of the great gurus of partnership and now one of our most loyal supporters and mentors. The Chicago connection doesn't stop there. Ann Clark, a classmate of mine from college, dragooned her small architecture firm and family into redesigning the hospital plans. Under Marjorie's leadership, they all rallied donors and companies to the cause, building a powerful "community of concern" in Chicagoland. A former construction company owner from Boston, Jim Ansara, had been advising reconstruction efforts since the quake and was ready to pour time and resources and connections into making this one bigger and better. Together, this crew revised the plans more than a dozen times, enlarging their scope again and again, and making it, in the end, a 205,000-square-foot, 320-bed medical center. That was three times the size of anything we'd ever attempted to build before. Let's say that these plans were our response to inveterate failures of imagination.

When I visited it last month, the Mirebalais Hospital sprawled across a small dell like a temple, gleaming white and girdled by black Haitian ironwork. To see, in the largest city on the Central Plateau, an elegant hospital and medical campus taking shape across what was once a bit of broken terrain running from steep conical hills down to an unproductive rice paddy would be a stirring image for any visitor. But it is especially moving for anyone who remembers the modest and often discouraging beginnings of Partners In Health a few hundred yards down the road almost thirty years ago.

The Mirebalais Hospital has also introduced new technologies into Haiti's public sector: it's the largest solar-powered hospital in the developing world. It has created hundreds of jobs, many of them permanent. Although we can't take direct credit, we're proud of the efflorescence of hotels, small businesses, beauty shops, and other micro-enterprises around Partners In Health–affiliated hospitals. The people we serve don't yet have jobs in the generative sector beyond agriculture. But release them from the burden of disease as a first step, and they will.

To some, the hospital is just a building in progress, one project among many. But for me it's emblematic of our respect for the Haitian people and of our aspiration to make the fruits of science and the art of healing more readily available to people in sore need of them.

III.

How does this story relate to you graduates who head off into the world today? First, try to *counter failures of imagination*. A great many people, including public health experts and some of our own coworkers, shook their heads and advised against the more ambitious version of the Mirebalais Hospital. I'm not saying they were wrong. It will be a long time before we can declare this effort a success. Hospitals are the bedrock of every health system, but they are large, expensive, complex institutions to run. The complexity of hospital-based care is one of the reasons public health starts with the low-hanging fruit: vaccines, family planning, prenatal care, bednets, hand washing, and latrines.

But the more difficult health and development problems—from drug-resistant tuberculosis, mental illness, and cancer to lack of education, clean water, roads, and food security—cannot simply be left for a better day. What about the higher-hanging fruit? Do the tools and strategies of global health permit us to care for people with more complex afflictions? Can we answer more of the need?

The short answer: of course we can, with innovation and resolve and a bolder vision than has been registered over the several decades.

Second point: as you seek to imagine or reimagine solutions to the greatest problems of our time, *harness the power of partnership.*

Partnership has been the font of our work since it began in Mirebalais three decades ago. It's why we refer to our collective as *Partners* In Health in a dozen languages. Sometimes, these are partnerships among service providers, teachers, and researchers. Always they are partnerships among people from very different backgrounds (within one country or across many). Sometimes the partnerships link different sorts of medical expertise—surgical, medical, psychiatric, and so on. Sometimes they bring together people who design and build hospitals with those who know how to power them with renewable energy or link them to the information grid. Sometimes they link talented students around the globe, as we've learned from organizations like GlobeMed, founded right here at Northwestern. Above all, such partnerships link those who can serve with those who need services—and seek to bring the latter group into the former, by recruiting them to act as community health workers, for example. By moving people from "patient" to "provider" and from "needy" to "donor," we can help break the cycle of poverty and disease. That's our sustainability model.

Partnerships are not always easy to maintain. Often competition rules when collaboration should prevail. People working to fight poverty are, like my doctor-friend in Mirebalais decades ago, too often schooled for scarcity. Where joblessness is the status quo, building new hospitals and schools can bring disappointment to some: everyone wants to work there—and usually not because they want a better job, but because they want a job, period. If someone else gets a job, our colleagues assume that they will not.

This sort of limited-good, zero-sum thinking is to be expected among those living in poverty, who know from first-hand experience that good things usually are in short supply. But such thinking is less acceptable among goodwill groups (foreign or homegrown) and among development experts seeking to attack poverty. Poverty will not surrender to a zero-sum strategy. And neither will the other great challenges before us, from global warming to prolonged and equitable growth of the world's economy.

Remember, graduates, that your own success will not come without real partnership. Do not think of it as coming at the cost of someone else's success. As new challenges arise to the survival of all dwellers on this planet, your generation, more than any other, will need to embrace partnership. So when you go out and paint that rock, do it together.

President Schapiro, friends and family, Chicagoland community of concern, and especially you, Class of 2012, thank you for having me back to Northwestern.

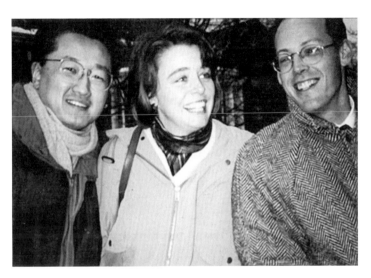

Figure 1. Partners In Health founders, Jim Yong Kim, Ophelia Dahl, and Paul Farmer, met for the first time in 1983. They have, together and with the help of many others, grown the organization from its initial work in a squatter settlement in rural Haiti. Today Partners In Health works in twelve countries around the world. Credit: Partners In Health.

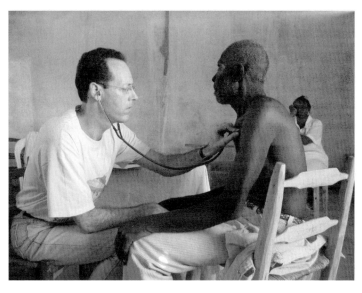

Figure 2. Paul Farmer joins mobile clinic, central Haiti, 2002. Credit: Mark Rosenberg.

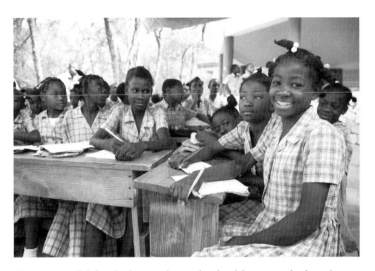

Figure 3. It didn't take long to learn that health care and education are complementary endeavors. Today, Partners In Health tries to link the delivery of health services with programs that seek to protect the social and economic rights of our patients and their families. Credit: Martha Adams.

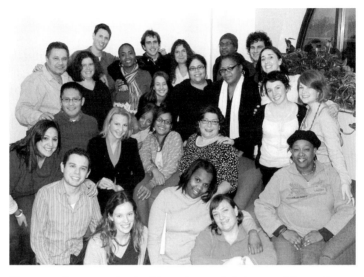

Figure 4. A community health worker model pioneered in rural Haiti has proven effective in treating chronic disease in hard-up neighborhoods in the United States since the mid-1990s. Dr. Heidi Behforouz (center) leads the Boston-based Prevention and Access to Care and Treatment (PACT) program. Credit: PACT.

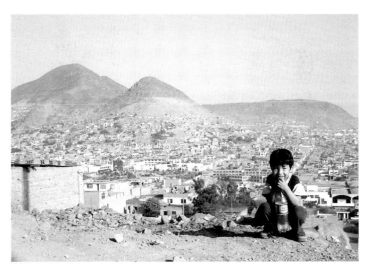

Figure 5. All around Lima, Peru's capital city replete with sky-
scrapers and colonial architecture, are informal settlements called
invasiones. It is in these poor neighborhoods that multidrug-resistant
tuberculosis has taken its greatest toll. Partners In Health has worked
with Peruvian authorities and many local tuberculosis specialists
since the mid-1990s to help bring the epidemic to heel. Credit: Socios
En Salud.

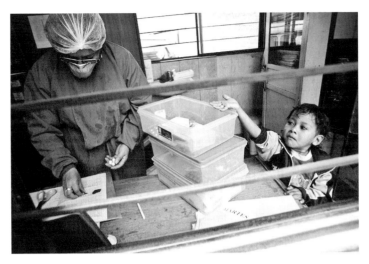

Figure 6. Socios En Salud, Partners In Health's sister organization in Peru, has worked with affected families and communities to help develop platforms for the management of drug-resistant tuberculosis, which requires both clinical acumen and delivery capacity. Credit: Enrique Castro-Mendivil.

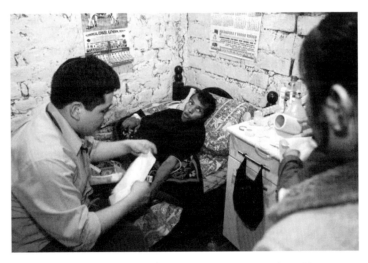

Figure 7. Although young people are among those affected by highly drug-resistant strains of tuberculosis, they can almost always be treated. Partners In Health has tried to make sure that Socios En Salud and its partners in the Ministry of Health have all the tools (diagnostics and drugs) needed to treat some of Peru's sickest patients. Credit: Socios En Salud.

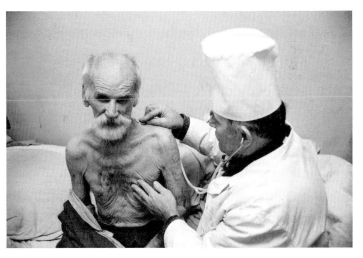

Figure 8. A Russian tuberculosis specialist examines a prisoner-patient in Tomsk (Siberia), 1999. Tuberculosis was far and away the leading cause of death not only among elderly prisoners but also among young men and women detained. Prison staff, including clinicians, were also afflicted. Photo credit: Partners In Health.

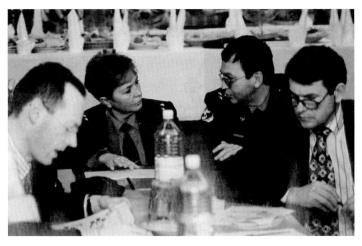

Figure 9. Paul Farmer and colleagues from Russia's justice ministry and the U.S. Centers for Disease Control and Prevention review laboratory data relevant to clinical efforts on behalf of prisoners with tuberculosis, 1999. Credit: Sergei Gitman.

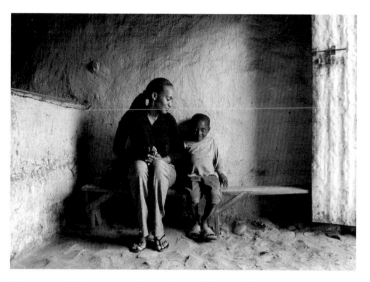

Figure 10. A Rwandan social worker visits a pediatric patient. Accompaniment is the heart of Partners In Health. Credit: Ilvy Njiokiktjien.

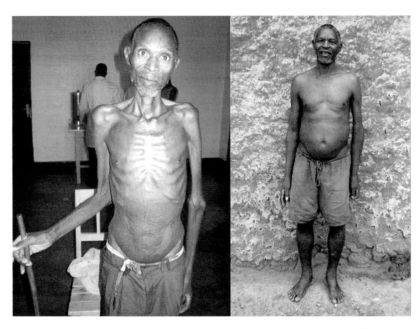

Figure 11. John, diagnosed with "terminal AIDS" in 2005, had, in fact, early HIV disease, extrapulmonary tuberculosis, and malnutrition. He thus needed three interventions: treatment for AIDS, tuberculosis, and hunger. The next photo shows how well he did—so well, perhaps, as Paul Farmer and he later joked that "he went from looking like Skeletor to looking like someone who needed Lipitor." Credit: Inshuti Mu Buzima.

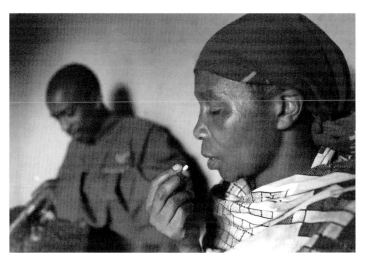

Figure 12. As fewer people in Rwanda are affected by AIDS, tuberculosis, malaria, and death in childbirth, other chronic diseases have emerged as a ranking challenge. Partners In Health seeks to build, in conjunction with the Rwandan health ministry and other partners, systems capable of delivering medications and services regularly in order to keep an aging population healthy. Credit: Matthieu Zellweger.

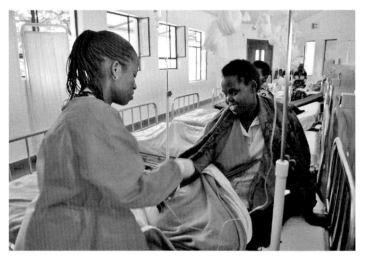

Figure 13. Cancer treatment in rural Africa is not impossible, as has been sometimes argued; it requires adequate infrastructure and a quorum of qualified providers. (There is no scarcity of patients.) This model has been embraced by the Rwandan Ministry of Health, Partners In Health, the Clinton Health Access Initiative, the Dana Farber Cancer Institute, Brigham and Women's Hospital, and the Jeff Gordon Children's Foundation in Butaro. Credit: Aubrey Davis

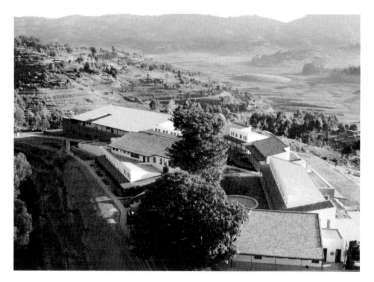

Figure 14. Butaro hospital is the only public hospital in northern Rwanda's Burera district, home to nearly 400,000 souls. Built by Partners In Health for the Rwandan health ministry, it is a public-private partnership for health equity. Central Africa's first cancer treatment center was launched here in mid-2012. Credit: Inshuti Mu Buzima.

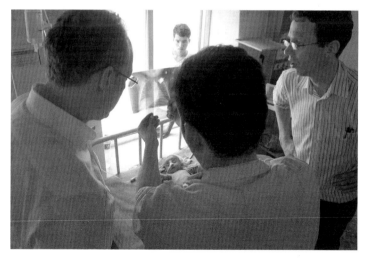

Figure 15. In rural, far-western Nepal, which has little in the way of modern health services, a number of Paul Farmer's former trainees have launched a health equity program. One of them, Duncan Mauru (right), studies a baby's X-ray with Paul (left) and his Nepali associate, Uday Kshatriya, in 2012. Credit: Rebecca Rollins.

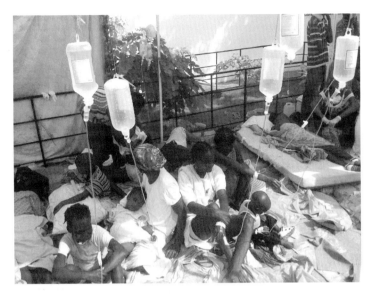

Figure 16. Haiti was ill prepared for the first cholera epidemic documented on its shores in at least a century. No one should die from cholera, which can in most cases be treated with simple rehydration. Photo credit: David Darg.

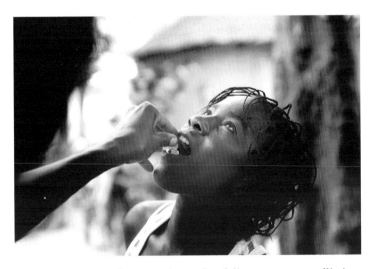

Figure 17. Accompaniment can be used to deliver treatment, palliation, and cure; it can also be powerful in the press for prevention. A young girl in Bocozel, Haiti, receives one of the Western Hemisphere's first doses of cholera vaccine, June 2012. Credit: Jonathan Lascher.

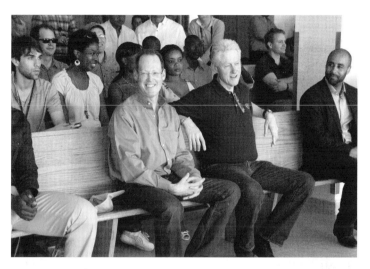

Figure 18. Paul Farmer, President Bill Clinton, and David Walton, the first graduate of the global health residency program at Harvard, at the recently completed Mirebalais National Teaching Hospital, the most ambitious health infrastructure project in Haiti completed since the January 2010 earthquake. The Mirebalais Hospital is the largest solar-powered hospital in the developing world. Credit: Rebecca Rollins.

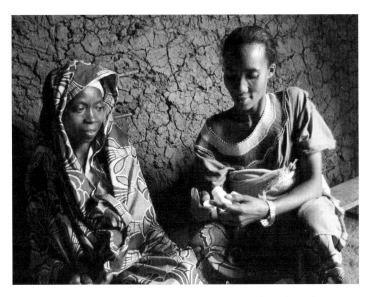

Figure 19. Photographer Laurie Wen has captured, perhaps better than anyone, the intimate and indispensible exchange between a Rwandan patient and her accompagnateur. Credit: Laurie Wen.

PART II

The Future of Medicine and the Big Picture

The speeches in Part II explore the same equity challenges as the last section but are directed to members of the medical community, and especially to newly minted physicians. This is a group of people about to spend almost all of their waking hours caring for patients, usually in teaching hospitals and affiliated clinics. I would make the same remarks to any providers of clinical care—including nurses, psychologists, social workers, and community health workers.

These comments convey three main messages.

First, physicians have a hard time seeing the *big picture*, the large-scale social forces that so often determine who gets sick and who has access to care. Doctors and service providers in general are trained to care for individual patients in clinics and hospitals, away from their families and communities. But always it is social and economic forces that dictate why and how the patients in front of us have come to be there in the first place. Public health specialists have long leveled this critique at clinical medicine, and all doctors and nurses would do well to pay attention.[1]

Moreover, medical professionals too often see our patients from the point of view of our specialty and our specialty alone. When you're a hammer, the saying goes, everything looks like a nail. I learned this lesson—and a related proverb—as a medical student practically living in a big Harvard teaching hospital. We medical students often found ourselves staying behind after a team of doctors had left the room, trying to explain diagnoses and treatment plans to patients and their families. This was harder, I learned, than translating from one language to another because every sub-specialty medical service seemed to see patients and their problems in a different way. I once complained about this to the resident leading our team. "Ask a pizza man what's for dinner," he observed with a smile, "and he'll tell you pizza."

The big picture isn't a pizza or a nail but rather an honest understanding of what causes premature suffering, what can be done to palliate it, with what tools old and new, and by whom. This press for comprehensiveness is the task of *social medicine*. I learned from my teachers that a physician's own experience and training and professional choices seldom lead to a reliable understanding of the patient's world. We must all strive to understand the social worlds in which our patients live, get sick, and seek care.

Second, the relationship between provider and patient affords an intimacy despite the social disparities one sees in a hospital, whether in Boston or in Haiti. Caregiving brings with it great privilege. It isn't just defined as saving lives or palliating suffering, nor is it solely performed by physicians. As my mentor Arthur Kleinman points out in his most recent writings, the majority of the caregiving that goes on in the world is administered not by doctors or nurses but by families and communities.[2]

The majority of this unpaid and underappreciated labor comes from mothers, sisters, aunts, and daughters.[3] Linking technical competence to caregiving and compassion and, sometimes, to consolation is the central task of good medicine.

Third, delivery matters. This may seem too obvious to be worth mentioning in a commencement speech. But study after study has shown that even in the United States, where these speeches were given, mediocrity and medical error and systemic flaws are too frequent. High-quality medical care often fails to reach those who need it most. We have centers of excellence, but we also have a long way to go before we bring quality care to scale. That's why many of my colleagues, including Jim Yong Kim, have been advocating for a "science of health care delivery."[4] The word "science" may be overly grand; a codification of best practices would be a step in the right direction. The extraordinary promise of modern medicine will remain unmet until the sickest patients receive care of the highest possible quality.

If You Take the Red Pill:
Reflections on the Future
of Medicine

Harvard Medical School, Class Day

JUNE 5, 2003

Giving graduation speeches, I've discovered, is in ways akin to what we all went through second year, when we first really listened to case presentations: there are ground rules for what is said and what is not, but one isn't sure exactly what they are. And just when you've mastered the sort of presentation appropriate to one medical specialty, you end up on a surgery team wondering, why all those withering glances during rounds when one begins, innocently enough, with "Mrs. Jones is a left-handed 57-year-old with seasonal allergies and a remote history of eczema, who now presents with hypotension and splenic rupture after an MVA"?[5]

So it is with graduation speeches. Worse, these talks often border on the absurd. Absurd and boring because parents and other family members—known in medicine as "insignificant others"—are not all that interested in the arcane details of medicine, much less speculation regarding its future. With the exception of those of you who are the children of doctors, you know your family has no clue, really, what you've just spent four years doing. Most of your kin also have no clue what you're in for next, but that's the subject of my talk today: the future of medicine, our own future.

Such speeches are also often absurdly irrelevant because the graduates, quite naturally, have every intention of marking this great rite of passage with serious revelry that's likely to damage short-term memory.

As if these were not serious enough handicaps—the mysterious rules of what can and cannot be said, the need to use age-specific insider speech and still avoid boring our guests, and the likelihood that substantial portions of today's activities will be forgotten by morning—there is another one. Inviting me to speak is perilous because, as a graduate of Harvard Medical School thirteen years ago, I do in fact know what you've been through, old school though HMS may have been back then. And I've had the immense good fortune of serving on this faculty during each one of those years since. So we've actually *shared* many of these experiences, putting parents and others at even greater risk of exclusion.

Look, your other insignificant others, including those who've footed the astronomical bills for your medical education, are already fidgeting. "He's going to be boring," they're thinking. "He's going to say technical things we won't understand." And some of the senior faculty, my own teachers, may have other concerns. "We know this guy. He's going to violate the unwritten rules of graduation speaking and offend someone, a major donor, say, or a really conservative parent."

Some of those fears may be justified. But I won't offend anyone for two reasons. First, I finally found, with the help of one of the amazing reference librarians at Countway, the complete set of rules regarding what can and cannot be said during graduation speeches.[6] I spent the last month reviewing these tomes, which weighed as much as if they'd been written by OSHA or a team of French philosophers.[7]

I took to heart the major ground rules. Indeed, I found this 24-volume set of commencement speech rules very helpful. Volume 16, Chapter 39, contains a long section, not yet on MEDLINE, regarding the exceptions made for medical school commencement speeches. Although post-eighteenth-century religion and politics remain forbidden topics, I learned that it's perfectly acceptable to talk about the future of medicine and even to dip into science, epidemiology, and health policy. Medical ethics, surveys say, is also fair game.

I further learned, in Volume 7, Chapter 12, that the size of the institution's endowment is inversely proportional to the degree to which the speaker must suck up to major donors during the speech itself. In the happy instance that the institution is financially secure, I read, one may address the students directly. So, having conferred with university accountants regarding the good financial health of HMS, I'll be talking today to you young doctors.

As for the other rules, which range from who may be quoted and who may not, the rules on religion and politics are clear: out of the question, states Chapter 19 of Volume 1. And the eighteenth-century clause is now being revised, with many arguing that the prohibition be pushed back to include the Crusades, which in the past two years have also been stricken from the list of acceptable commencement topics in the heartlands and in less financially secure institutions. But I'd already decided not to talk much about world politics. It's too confusing for us doctors. As the great American philosopher Chris Rock put it recently, "You know the world is going crazy when the best rapper is a white guy, the best golfer is a black guy, the Swiss hold the America's Cup, France is accusing the United States of arrogance, and Germany doesn't want to go to war."

Best to stick to medicine. But then there are three entire volumes in the series exhorting the speaker not to be boring, to seek culturally relevant and age-appropriate referents. And not just any will do, according to Volume 4, Chapter 32. The Dixie Chicks are out. And Eminem, I just learned, has been stripped of the Good Speech-giving Seal of Approval and no longer appears at all in *Bartlett's Book of Quotations.*

I.

To return to my opaque title, "If You Take the Red Pill." If my research is sound, almost all the graduates here today know that I am not talking about a vitamin or about the stool softener, colace. It was the same Countway librarian, in fact, who showed me data suggesting that fully 94.2 percent of the Class of 2003 have seen *The Matrix.* And I was impressed to learn, from the same authoritative source, that an impressive 47 percent of you have already seen *The Matrix Reloaded.* (A freakish 7 percent of you have seen this new film "five or more times," and may wish to confer with your classmates who have elected to pursue careers in psychiatry, should this obsession persist.)

In any case, most of you young doctors smiled knowingly as you looked at your programs and noted the title of my speech. My sources also say that, although the Dean has not himself seen these or any other action movies in recent years, he is looking at me with affectionate tolerance, rather than the tense anxiety that may have clouded the fair features of some of his predecessors. As I said, he knows I'll behave. (As an aside, note that I have full clearance to call him "Joe," because he doesn't like to be called "Dean Martin."[8] Granted, it's not a distinguished image, that of a tipsy entertainer from a group known as the "Rat Pack." But then again it's not like his parents named him "Dean." He was doing just fine, a famous neurologist, and, boom, he goes and becomes a dean.)

In any case, one last word to those unfamiliar with my reference to *The Matrix*. It's an action film starring that great thespian, Keanu Reeves. The plot is murky but not uninteresting: his character is a cog in the great wheel of industry and finance, just another programmer working in front of his computer screen in a gray cubicle. Lives in a big city, looks like Chicago or Toronto. Mr. Anderson, as he is called, knows something is very wrong with the world but doesn't know what it is. It's "like a splinter in his mind." There's got to be more to life than this, he's certain. He feels most alive under a different alias, his hacker name, Neo. To make a convoluted story short, Neo is contacted by a certain Morpheus, someone the company drones and police term a terrorist. Morpheus is played in completely over-the-top fashion by Laurence Fishburne. If Neo wants to find out what's bugging him—all the mediocrity and meaninglessness of life in the machine—then he, the fellow named Morpheus, will be only too happy to show him.

Before I get serious, I have to caution those among you who have not seen *The Matrix*, all seven of you out there: do not watch this self-important movie—which has already spawned dozens of scholarly books and seminars—with irreverent people. I made the mistake of seeing it with my sisters who maintained a parallel narrative throughout the film. For example, when Morpheus contacts Neo with a cell phone that rings seconds after arriving, via FedEx, Neo-Keanu answers, rather dully, "Hullo?"

"Do you know who this is?" asks Morpheus in grandiloquent fashion.

A long pause ensues, plenty long enough for my sisters to chime, in unison, "Laurence Fishburne, duh!"

But if you manage to avoid such rude if hilarious company, you'll have to admit that the plot line is a good one. And relevant to the world we inhabit.

Neo hooks up with Morpheus, of course. And Morpheus offers Neo a choice: he can choose to see the world as it really is, to extract that splinter from his mind. Or he can chicken out. Morpheus outlines Neo's choice with all the subtlety of a mediocre Shakespearean actor who's had a few too many vodka tonics. Morpheus pulls a pillbox out of his stylin' leather coat. He proffers a red pill and a blue pill. (And no, this is not the blue pill of interest to our senior faculty and to Pfizer stockholders.) Morpheus says something like this: "You take the blue pill, the story ends, you wake up in your bed and believe whatever you want to believe. You take the red pill, you remain in Wonderland and I show you how deep the rabbit hole goes."

Like any good action hero with a splinter in his mind, Neo goes for truth, which is all that Morpheus promises. And the truth is ugly. It's that Neo, and indeed everyone he's ever known, is a slave. Never mind, just now, what the mechanism of their enslavement is. I don't want to spoil the surprise for the seven of you who haven't yet seen the movie. The message is clear: Neo's been duped, deluded by job security and certain material comforts like cool club music and hip garb. It's all fake.

II.

It's my contention, of course, that a certain amount of red-pill popping is just what we need in medicine and public health. But how many of us want to see how deep the rabbit hole goes? (Returning to the rules of graduation speechmaking, I hasten to add that Lewis Carroll does not figure on the proscribed list of authors, at least not in Volume 3, which forbids quoting Shakespeare, Eminem, Kahlil Gibran, Flaubert—or in fact anyone French—or poetry by Tupac. Tupac's *lyrics*, on the other hand, are approved for graduation addresses in both physics and philosophy, and his work is widely cited at MIT and in the wild and crazy HST ceremonies to occur later this evening.)[9]

Do we dare take the red pill? A serious question from a guy who is gagging on the red pill and still falling down the rabbit hole. As a character in the film says—he's a bad guy, of course—"Ignorance is bliss."

But ignorance is not bliss. Ignorance is just that—ignorance—and ignorance and medicine are simply not compatible. Our own red pill may well be more bitter than any other, because it's easy to argue that, for doctors, as for scientists, the blue pill is an unacceptable option, even if it's what most of us have swallowed.

Gagging, I just said. Still falling. How so? This is your day, not mine, but your invitation meant an awful lot to me. In order to be here today, I traveled from rural Haiti to Boston via Moscow, where yesterday afternoon I brooded about my remarks and reviewed my notes on Volumes 11–26 of the Rule Book. And tomorrow I'm headed to Rwanda via Knoxville, Tennessee; it's not a direct flight. Then back to Haiti; but after ten days, I'm to be back in Africa. You've all heard of the New York shuttle. Well, I've been taking the Harvard-Haiti shuttle for 20 years, and I can tell you, it gets old. One starts hoping to come across a blue pill in those paltry bags of airplane peanuts, which currently constitute 32 percent of my entire dietary intake.

What's all this frenetic travel about? It's about the red pill. Honest. It's not that taking the truth pill leads you to board either hovercraft or airplane. It's rather that if you take it and you're a doctor, you see that there's unnecessary sickness and suffering everywhere on this planet. You see too that certain epidemics are completely out of control and that there are horrific health emergencies in each of the places I've just mentioned. You see that some people are denied access to the most basic fruits of science, to the tools developed over the past few decades as medicine itself earned its name as "the youngest science."

I'm an infectious disease doc, so of course I'm going to talk about epidemics. You think SARS is bad, and it is. But allow me to put this latest epidemic in perspective. As of today, although fewer than a thousand people have died of SARS, several Fortune 500 companies are scrambling to put together a global SARS fund; I'm told that hundreds of millions of dollars have been pledged. I just read that certain airports in Asia have installed thermal scanners to identify febrile travelers. All this in the space of a couple months. All good.

But over 8,000 people die *every day* of AIDS, the leading infectious cause of death in the modern world. And many more die of tuberculosis and malaria: during the course of this year, the year you graduate, six million people, most of them children and young adults, will die of these three diseases alone. Six million deaths, almost all of them preventable with modern medicine, but the red pill reminds us that we have no plan in place to serve those most in need. And even the newspapers, whose editors and publishers seem to subsist on a steady diet of blue pills, report that the Global Fund to Fight AIDS, Tuberculosis and Malaria will soon run out of money. The plagues of the poor don't seem to interest industry, the press, or even basic science.

So it is everywhere. Take the red pill and suddenly you see that 40 million Americans have no health insurance and as many more are poorly insured. Take the red pill and you see that the bottom billion of this planet don't have enough food or clean water while in other places, including this country, we are called to subsidize agribusiness and then destroy excess crops or dump them on faltering peasant economies, so delivering their coup de grâce. Take the red pill and you wonder why it is that, in the global era of connectivity, millions die of hunger while others battle obesity. You learn that some companies short-date perfectly good medications and equipment in a process known as "planned obsolescence" while tens of millions will die without ever having benefitted from the discoveries of Salk or Sabin or even Pasteur.[10] This has been going on for some time in the *desert of the real,* and it's getting worse.

Why dredge up this dreary stuff on a day of celebration? Because you, members of the Class of 2003, can change all this. Indeed, you must. It's urgent. Sure, it's utopian, but it's also feasible. Here's a glass half full for you: as doctors, you are granted special license to fight for a better world. You can carp about health insurance in a way that politicians cannot, because you are merely fighting for your patients. You can gripe about drug prices in a way that others cannot, for the same reasons. You can even deliver a red-pill speech like this one without being considered a pill yourself.

Because this is what we're called to do: to fight for the survival and the dignity of our patients, especially the sickest and most vulnerable.

You don't have to travel far to meet people who receive substandard care. Some of you in this class have worked with our own group in a neighborhood less than a mile from here. Many students are astounded at how few of our patients in Roxbury have ever had a doctor visit them in their homes. But the red pill suggests that it's after the patients leave the hospital that many of them have troubles—troubles understanding or following doctors' orders. Troubles filling prescriptions. Troubles getting to clinic appointments. Troubles paying rent or utility bills.

You could address some of these troubles yourselves. Say you're an orthopedics resident and on the way from the gym to the hospital, you pop by and see the lady who fell and fractured her femoral neck. You helped to put in the hardware and all went splendidly, as you noted in your brief (very brief) op note. She lives on the fifth floor of a run-down public housing building not a mile from the medical mecca in which you train. The elevator's out. If you'd taken the blue pill, you wouldn't even know this fact, because she lives in the desert of the real, invisible, it would seem, to the majority of doctors.

Let's bring this back to earth, some of you may be thinking. After all, you weren't in Moscow yesterday and, with an exception or two, you're not headed to Haiti tomorrow. You're thinking instead about internship and beyond. It's a big change from medical school. Speaking for myself, I think residency is a wonderful time. I loved it. You're officially doctors as of today, but in a couple weeks you're going to be the only doctors some people have, period. Your patients will be counting on you.

A lot of people whine about internship. The hours are too long, they say. Well sure, being a doctor can be hard at three in the morning. But it's not as hard as being a patient. How difficult is it, really, to be a practitioner of modern biomedicine? On all these planes, I see the captains of industry looking very industrious. I'm usually reading *People* magazine and they're going through their spreadsheets. Do you think, really, that we work all that much harder than bankers or stockbrokers? I'm not convinced, frankly.

Rather, it's what we do that is so radically different. Whether internist or pediatrician or pathologist or cardiac surgeon, we are working for others. It's not about us, or our incomes, or our sense of personal efficacy. It's about what happens to our patients. Or, for those of you who are scientists, it's about the knowledge you create that can help heal a wounded world.

After a few 100-hour workweeks, there may be moments when you want to take the blue pill. Don't do it. Wonderful things are happening in clinical medicine and the allied sciences, in large part because of medicine's embrace of science. The yield of this embrace has been nothing short of marvelous. No branch of medicine has been untouched. From pathology to oncology to infectious disease, the revolution continues.

But for those who take the red pill, we are obliged to see the dark side of progress. More and better discoveries, every day, but an erosion in our ability to use them wisely and equitably. More capacity to engineer new therapies but a lack of commitment to directing our efforts toward the world's great killers. In my field, there have been many victories, certainly. But there hasn't been a new class of antituberculosis drug discovered in decades. As of June 2003, there are no effective vaccines for AIDS, TB, or malaria—the big three modern plagues.

Visits to the lifeworlds of the sick help us see how terribly behind we are in the equity arena. We're failures in the equity department. There are many reasons to visit patients in their homes: they help us understand why excellent in-hospital care can come to naught if we lack an equity plan. Visits help us understand why prescriptions go unfilled, why appointments are missed, why medications are taken incorrectly or not at all. Visits connect us to people whose lives are very different from our own.

This failure, which you can see for yourselves during internship and residency, is emblematic of the even more shocking failures one can see when one leaves behind nationality, a blue-pill side effect, and takes on the globe's medical problems. This brings me to a different, more personal part of the message—the dismount, you'll be glad to know.

III.

If you've agreed with me so far, then you'll see all the vast promise of modern medicine and also the dismal state of our global village. More and more for fewer and fewer. It's true in so many realms, but it's excruciatingly so in medicine and public health. I promised you I would not cite Shakespeare, since the rules forbid it, but Martin Luther King is credited with having said the following: "Of all the forms of inequality, injustice in health is the most shocking and the most inhumane."[11]

Taking the red pill is a scary process. There are those of you out there today who threw back the red pill but are now reaching for the ipecac. And who wouldn't be? We live in a world of medical haves and have-nots, a world in which most of the bottom billion have no modern medical care at all, a world in which current trends promise that the situation will get worse during the early years of your medical practice.

What are the boundaries of your world? Next year, they will shrink to a hospital or two, and all you'll want to do when you leave the hospital will be to watch an action film by yourself. Or listen to some music. Or do whatever it is that transports you out of the desert of the real. But in your heart, and in your practice, you know that most of the boundaries are ones we create ourselves. They're boundaries we erect in order to lessen *our* pain, not the pain of others.

Where exactly do you fit in? You are graduates from what is probably the finest medical school on the face of the globe, and you live in the global era. Since the Roman Empire existed well before the Crusades, it's OK to mention it without violating the rules and regulations laid down in Volume 2 of the graduation-speech code of honor. But let's face it: you're card-carrying members of the world's one superpower, the latter-day Rome. It doesn't matter all that much where you were born or to what circumstances: no other crop of young doctors will ever have the latitude and influence you will; no others have yet had the technology. Perhaps it's cheating to quote last month's *Harper's Magazine*. In an essay every American should read, William Finnegan writes

> The U.S. currently enjoys a truly rare global preeminence—military, economic, pop-cultural. But power is not, obviously, the same as legitimacy. And every over-weening, remorseless projection of American power, every unfair trade rule and economic double standard jammed into the global financial architecture, helps erode the legitimacy of American ascendancy in the eyes of the world's poor.[12]

"This erosion," concludes Finnegan, "is occurring throughout Latin America, Africa, Asia." I live and work in these places, and I know he's right. The future of medicine is also jammed into this global financial architecture. That's why our group in Haiti has had to fight tooth and nail to use the tools of modern biomedicine among the destitute sick, since they do not constitute "a market." That's why we develop thermal sensors for Asian business commuters while another febrile continent's rigors go uncharted.

If I conclude by saying things like "go forth and heal the world," I know you're going to groan. I'm regularly subjected to the gentle mockery of the second-year show.[13] Just so the parents here know what we mean, I will read from the program of the most recent show. In this "newspaper," a front-page item reads as follows:

Farmer Sells Kidney to Save Village

HAITI—Harvard Medical School professor Dr. Paul Farmer sold his second kidney yesterday to provide lifesaving tuberculosis medicines to a remote village near the Haitian capital of Port-au-Prince. . . . He felt it would be better to have a life of dialysis than lose another soul to this treatable disease. When asked about his courage, Dr. Farmer replied quite heroically, "So thirsty . . ."

All jest aside, though, taking the red pill and seeing the world of the sick as it is today leads us to painful choices. I'm not seeking to be Manichaean: the choices before you are not between good and bad. They're between doing good and doing better.

To do better, don't we have to take that red pill and fight?

Your generation is going to have to answer this question. Because unfortunately, as Morpheus says, you and I have run out of time. Of course, the clock isn't really ticking on us. It's ticking on others. Again—how many people have died of treatable diseases during the time it took for me to give this talk? Especially on that febrile continent to which I return tomorrow?

IV.

Allow me to leave you with two take-home messages, as we say at HMS.

First, apply the Golden Rule in your practice—especially during that last admission, in the wee hours of the morning. Or to a particularly difficult or crabby patient. Could you ever care as much about her as you do about, say, your own mother? Could you ever love someone as much as you love yourself or your own child? The answer to these questions may well be "certainly not," but at least the red pill pushes us to ask them.

Second, make home visits now and again. Don't buy the received wisdom about "respecting boundaries." What's wrong with helping housebound patients wash their dishes? Or helping hut-bound patients transform dirt floors into cement floors? Break down boundaries. Think outside the box. Do you want to wake up some day and discover that your life has become dim, without color? That you took the blue pill? Even though your ectopic soul, stowed away, say, in your left axilla, forgotten, neglected, was exhorting you all along to make the leap, to take a chance?

You know the questions. The answer is out there, and you will find it if you want to.

Now you know. And knowing, as another action figure was fond of noting, is half the battle.

And that, dear doctors and families and friends and colleagues and deans, concludes my speech. Thank you and congratulations, Class of 2003.

Medicine as a Vocation

University of Miami Miller School of Medicine,
Commencement

MAY 15, 2004

What better way to start and end a speech like this than to belt out a hearty congratulations? I'm here to serve up that bizarre admixture of cheerleading and avuncular advice that is the commencement speech. I feel lucky to be here because Miami has always loomed large in my life. I grew up in Hernando County, near Weeki Wachee, spring of live mermaids. Back then, Miami loomed large as the wild and crazy metropolis far to the south, the place we all wanted to visit—and would have except our parents even back then thought of St. Pete as far too wild and crazy a metropolis for kids from Hernando County.

But when you're old enough to vote, you're old enough to go to South Florida—although perhaps it's not polite to mention Florida's voting history in a graduation speech. In any case, I finally made that road trip to Miami while in college and have been coming back ever since.

In fact, I've been flying between Harvard and Haiti for more than two decades, and it's not a direct flight: Miami International Airport is my home away from home.

Miami is not only your home and my hub, though—it's the capital of the Americas. Everywhere I go in the broad world, I find that Miami means something. Someone in Rwanda asked me recently if I was a devotee of *CSI Miami*, and I didn't have a clue.

And of course Miami is a really big deal in Haiti, where I spend much of my time. Some of the people with whom I live in rural Haiti use the word "Miami" to stand for the "United States." When I'm headed back to Boston, they often say, "So you're off to Miami?" I just say yes. They're sure Harvard Medical School is situated in Miami, along with Disney World, the Pentagon, Hollywood, and pretty much everything of note north of the Spanish Main.

So my Haitian neighbors and patients, who have never heard of Yale or Brown, are now very proud that I am at last going to give a commencement speech in the city that matters. For the major props I'm getting in Haiti alone, I thank you for this invitation!

I. ON THE MEANING OF GRADUATION

My job today is to cheer you on and give you a little advice. In the eyes of some, my credentials in this arena are scant: I've not discovered any vaccines or genes, nor am I a dean or a department chair. But I *am* someone who loves not only Florida, hanging chads aside, but also medicine. From pathology to neurosurgery, I just love medicine. And you will too, if you don't already.

Some cynics would now ask, so what?

Look at the way our world is today, early twenty-first century. There's great beauty, but also violence and war and mayhem; there are epidemics that should never have happened and others that are spiraling out of control even as we sit here. There is goodness and there is greed and great abuse of power.

But medicine, if practiced the way your generation could practice it, should be a great and unmitigated force for good. When we hear the term "the professions," we think of many trades. But I think that we know, in our hearts, that medicine is, or should be, different from the rest of them. Medicine is a *vocation*.

(That would make UM an *awfully* expensive vocational school, is what your parents are thinking right now.)

Of course, it's also true that medicine can be twisted or even perverted, which is why Carl Hiaasen, himself a native of these parts, can write entertaining novels that are also instructive warnings, reminders of how we can all make mistakes. There are dark chapters in the annals of medicine, as you all know, far darker than in Hiaasen's novel.

As the new generation, it's your responsibility to see that bad things don't happen on your watch. Because as of today, my friends, you're legal. You're doctors. As we used to say at Harvard Medical School, which uses the pass/fail system, "P = MD."

According to Hiaasen, you're more legal here than in other places. If his novels are well researched—and I've a hunch they are—even an internist like me could practice plastic surgery in some settings in our state. Florida is, let's be honest, something of a rule-bending place.

One Hiaasen character is a plastic surgeon described in uncharitable terms: Dr. Rudy Graveline smiled when the Florida sun came out because "it baked and fried and pitted the facial flesh, and seeded the pores with vile microscopic cancers that would eventually sprout and require excision."[14] Since the good doctor was a graduate of Harvard Medical School, we know it's just fiction, right?

Right?

In the novel, something very bad—since we all just ate, let's just call it an irreversible medical error involving a lot of arterial blood—happens when Dr. G. performs liposuction to make a quick buck. It is, according to Hiaasen's novel,

> the most common cosmetic procedure performed in this country, with more than 100,000 operations a year. The mortality rate for suction-assisted lipectomy is relatively low, about one death for every 10,000 patients. The odds of complications—which include blood clots, fat embolisms, chronic numbness, and severe bruising—increase considerably if the surgeon performing the liposuction has had little or no training in the procedure. Rudy Graveline fell decisively into this category—a doctor who had taken up liposuction for the simple reason that it was exceedingly lucrative. No state law or licensing board or medical review committee required Rudy to study liposuction first, or become proficient, or even be tested on his surgical competence before trying it.... Rudy Graveline was a licensed physician, and legally that meant he could try any damn thing he wanted.
>
> He did not give two hoots about certification by the American Board of Plastic Surgery, or the American Academy of Facial Plastic and Reconstructive Surgery, or the American Society of Plastic and Reconstructive Surgeons. What were a couple more snotty plaques on the wall? His patients could care less. They were rich and vain and impatient.... Only a boor, white trash or worse, would ever question the man's techniques or complain about his results.[15]

Now, a boy from Weeki Wachee might take offense at Hiaasen's reference to white trash, but leave that aside. I will return to Dr. G. after I tell you a very different and true story about plastic surgery. I'll return to medical errors, too. But first let me ask you this: although choices are rarely stark, you will, once in a while, have to choose. What's it going to be? Medicine as a force for good or medicine as just another business?

II. ON WHAT YOU'VE DONE

I have ample reason to stand before you and answer that question with optimism and hope. And I'm speaking quite specifically to you, graduates and students and faculty of the University of Miami. My conviction comes from experience, because I've had the good fortune to work with some of you in Haiti.

Haiti's a very important place, especially here in Florida. Haiti is our oldest neighbor. It's one of Florida's top trading partners. Many Haitians live here in Miami, contributing to the economic and social life of this great metropolis. There are proud Haitian parents here today. Haiti's on my mind all the time, and I think of Haiti with great gratitude, because I've learned so much from the Haitian people. In fact, I don't know who made a mint on that book *Everything I Know I Learned in Kindergarten*, or whatever it's called, but I'm thinking about writing *Everything I Know I Learned in Haiti*. Granted, my teachers at Harvard would not be pleased with such a title, but I have a great debt to Haiti. That's where I learned what sort of medicine I wanted to practice. It's also where I came to understand how strange life's lottery can be. Why was I born over here rather than just an hour and a half away?

Growing up in Florida, I knew little about life's lottery. I knew so little about the history of either Florida or Haiti. When I was a kid in the Hernando County public school system, I don't believe I learned, for example, that the United States occupied Haiti militarily for two decades of the twentieth century. I don't think I even learned about the great slave revolt that made Haiti Latin America's first independent nation. I don't recall learning a thing about the indigenous people of that island, who are as gone as the Calusa people of Florida. Weeki Wachee was not always a tourist attraction but rather home to the people who named it: "Weeki Wachee" means "little spring" in the Muskogee language, and although I was not heedless of the great beauty of the place, I gave little thought to our state's troubled history.

We are sitting today in a place once peopled by the Calusa, who were called "the Fierce Ones" because they were the most powerful people in South Florida when the Spanish arrived in the sixteenth century. They were wiped out by smallpox, a gift from the Europeans, and also by wars and conquest—those also, gifts from the Europeans. The Calusa, we now read in the *Miami Herald*, "built large shell-mound settlements, most of which were torn down in the 20th century to be used as road fill or removed to make room for development."[16]

Doesn't that just kill you? *As road fill?*

Don't worry, I won't dwell on the past on commencement day. I'm going to return to the future, which is what concerns us now. But we all know the old saw about being condemned to repeat the past if we don't learn from it.

The truth of this old saw came to me after leaving Florida, when I was in college. Many of you here today know that you're lucky to be graduating from a great medical school. When I say "lucky" I'm not suggesting that you're not also hard-working, never shirk your reading, are always on time for rounds, and spend all your down time reading Harrison's or searching MED-LINE. Certainly, none of you would ever chill out when the sick, wherever they are, might be made better or even cheered up. But seriously, aren't we all a bit lucky to have ended up here and not, say, in a drought-stricken village somewhere in Africa? Or in a war-torn settlement somewhere in the Middle East? A drug-riven "outsourced" neighborhood in one of this nation's large cities?

So I hope it's OK for me to ask, how has awareness of our good fortune informed your choices so far? Well, all of you have chosen a career in medicine, a healing art that is based, increasingly, on science. And I've had firsthand experience of your goodwill. Some people here today were part of the very first neurosurgical operations ever performed in rural Haiti: they were done in Cange, in the hospital of which I am co–medical director. And many more of you have been to the town of Thomonde, where Medishare and this university have breathed new life into the meaning of solidarity between our two countries, the two oldest republics in this hemisphere.

One member of your class helped organize a team of Miami plastic surgeons who, unlike Dr. Graveline, came to a squatter settlement in Haiti's central plateau to repair cleft palates among adults. Can you imagine what it's like to go through your whole life with an unrepaired defect like that? Here in the States, such surgery happens during childhood in order to spare children the psychological and social fallout of deformity. But the artistry of the UM plastic surgeons, and also that of the students who helped organize this work, was in this instance offered to adults. I marveled at the results, which were excellent. Cosmesis achieved, and without liposuction. But later I was talking to a student from Harvard Medical School who'd taken a fifth year to work in central Haiti and had referred half the cleft palate cases. I wanted a sense of how the patients had responded to this major change.

"What's life like for them now?" I asked. "I mean, 30 years

with a cleft palate and suddenly, boom!—you're beautiful. It must be really wonderful?"

David, an experienced Haiti hand, paused before answering. "To be frank," he replied, "they haven't focused that much on their newfound beauty. Don't get me wrong," he said. "They're grateful. But they're really a lot more concerned about where their next meal is coming from, how they're going to send their kids to school, the usual stuff."

The usual stuff. He was right, of course. I'd seen it before there and elsewhere—young adults dying of AIDS, weighing 70 pounds, who'd later double their body weight after a year on antiretrovirals (ARVs). As soon as they stopped dying, they too were more concerned about being able to make ends meet for their families than about their good medical care. They needed, still need, jobs and food and decent housing.

Does this mean we should cancel the cleft palate repairs? Does it mean we should replace ARV orders with plans to build factories or buy food?

Of course it doesn't. It means that we live in a world of horrible inequalities and we are called to do something, as doctors and as humans, to repair the world. The world itself has been cleft, and you are the surgeons who can have a hand in fixing it.

I guess this is my first bit of advice, which is more like pleading. You've got to do a better job than we have to date. I am not the sort of guy to ask you to all hold hands and sing "Kumbaya," but a big dose of healing is badly needed. Our world, the world of which Miami is far more a capital city than is Tallahassee, is a world cleft in two: the haves and the have-nots.

We're the haves. The rest of the world, or at least its bottom billion, are so busy with the hard business of survival that they don't have time to look in a mirror after a cleft palate repair. Some of them have never seen a mirror.

III. ON WHAT YOU'LL DO:
A BIT OF ADVICE

Graduation speeches should be short, and I'd love to close with something Churchillian, such as, "Go forth and face the world unflinchingly." But instead, let me give you more practical advice: always wear sunscreen.

Seriously though, I do want to end with some advice. Some of it may seem banal. It might surprise you when I advise you all to always keep studying. Technical competence is the least we can offer our patients.

How well are we doing? Perhaps Hiaasen's books are meant to make us laugh, but medical error remains an enormous problem, in spite of all the progress made.

Earlier this week, the RAND Corporation released expanded results from the largest and most comprehensive study of health care quality in the United States ever conducted. The study, published in the journal *Health Affairs*, shows that on average, residents of twelve U.S. communities receive between 50 and 60 percent of recommended care for acute and chronic conditions, and key preventive services, with little variation across diverse communities. According to the authors, these findings are consistent with decades of research that demonstrates sizable deficits in the quality of health care.[17]

I'm standing in front of hundreds of people and will make a confession: I still make little flash cards in order to learn about new diseases and new medicines. I still study, if not quite as assiduously as I did when a medical student. Medicine is the newest science, and the least we can do for our patients is to be more competent than some of the clowns in Hiaasen's novels.

In other places, including some close by, it's not that patients receive the wrong sort of care, but rather that they receive none at all. And so the rest of the advice I'll give you concerns the future of our vocation. A lot of you will stay right here in Florida; others will move around the globe, ending up, as I did, in unexpected places. But it matters less and less, in this age, where you live. If I had my druthers, I'd stay close by these parts. You've got the Everglades and Coconut Grove and the Parrot Jungle. You have *CSI Miami*. You have great cultural events. The last time I was here traffic was backed up because of a Britney Spears concert. But it doesn't matter all that much where you choose to live or what branch of medicine to practice: if you have faith in medicine as a vocation, you can make something great out of whatever it is you choose to do.

If you do stay here in South Florida, remember your classmates and teachers who are doing things like repairing cleft palates or supporting community health in central Haiti. Help them out. Or support projects for people living with spinal cord injuries who still want to learn to sail a boat. Or people who are sick but don't have insurance or even a place to live.

Try to make your medical practice move between the big picture and the small picture. By "small" I don't mean unimportant. Far from it. I mean the person at hand. The single suffering patient in front of you. I think anthropology taught me the importance of listening, but it's been in clinical medicine that this skill is most helpful. What sort of problems might a patient have filling a prescription or getting to an appointment? These are things you'll only discover by listening. Have you ever gone and bought groceries for a housebound patient? Have you ever washed their dishes when it's hard for them to stand at a sink, if they, unlike our patients in Haiti, have a sink? Science is what will make medicine truly powerful, but being humble and persistent is what makes medicine a vocation.

And keep the big picture in mind, too. What is the Big Picture, anyway? According to the Academy—the Academy of Motion Pictures, that is—the Big Picture this year was *The Return of the King.* Allow me draw your attention instead to the previous movie in the trilogy. There's a great speech in *The Two Towers.* It comes from the mouth of the humble and persistent Sam Gamgee, who, when asked if he's the hero's bodyguard, retorts, "No, his gardener."

Here's the speech, more or less. It's the movie's peroration, and it will be mine:

"It's all wrong," says Sam. "By rights we shouldn't be here, but we are. But it's like in the great stories, the ones that really mattered. Full of darkness and danger they were. And sometimes you didn't want to know the ending, because how could the end be happy? How could the world go back to the way it was when so much bad has happened?"

Here we are, in a world stained by slavery and sickness, by the destruction of the Calusa people and the degradation of their material culture into landfill. A world in which AIDS, tuberculosis, and malaria alone will this year kill six million people, most of them young adults and children. A world of war and real terrorism and also a place where we're keeping two-year-old Haitians locked up as "terror threats."

It's a world full of suffering, as any doctor who looks at the big picture knows. You'll want to hang up your hat sometimes. But the humble and persistent Sam continues: "Folk in those stories had a lot of chances of turning back, only they didn't. They were holding on to something."

"What are we holding on to, Sam?" asks the protagonist.

Sam doesn't hesitate in answering: "That there's some good in this world, and it's worth fighting for."

Class of 2004. Dear doctors, faculty, deans, alums, President Shalala.[18] There is good in this world, and it's worth fighting for. So what if you can't work 37 miracles in whatever time is accorded you? There's so much you *can* do, humbly, persistently. Just practicing medicine can be a quiet miracle.

Even Sam ends on a positive note, predicting that "a new day will come. And when the sun shines it'll shine out the clearer." So wear that sunscreen, and make modern medicine live up to its promise. Keep your patients and their problems in the forefront of your mind as much as you possibly can, but spend a little time, at least a little time, thinking about the big picture. Our troubled world calls for nothing less.

It's a tall order, I'll grant you. But humble persistence might just win the day.

Thank you, and good luck and congratulations to you and yours.

Haiti After the Earthquake

Harvard Medical School,
Talks@Twelve Speaker Series

FEBRUARY 11, 2010

As I left Boston to join my family in Haiti for the holidays, it did not occur to me that I would not be back here until today. I would like to express my gratitude, our gratitude, for the outpouring of support that has followed the earthquake that occurred one month ago tomorrow. That now seems like years ago, not days, but regardless, it is time to take stock of what happened and what is likely to happen in the coming months and years.

On the afternoon of January 12, one of our colleagues, a Harvard infectious disease specialist originally from Dublin and long working with Partners In Health, was in a meeting in Port-au-Prince as five o'clock approached. The meeting was about, of all things, disaster preparedness. Here is what Dr. Louise Ivers described:

> By Saturday, approximately five operating rooms were functional in the city, but the majority of injuries that I cared for in the first

---

Parts of this speech were adapted and published in *Haiti After the Earthquake* (New York: PublicAffairs, 2011).

few hours and days of the tragedy were open fractures and crush injuries that require antibiotics that we did not have. And surgery that we could not perform. With the help of surgeons who had just arrived, 48 hours after I found him on the street where we had both escaped with our lives from cracking buildings, we amputated the arm of a young man on a table in the open air with no available anaesthesia. Not to do so would have left him to die of gangrene.

Three days later, after flying over a city plunged in total darkness—only small fires and tiny spots of light illuminated the vast conurbation of Port-au-Prince, a city of three million souls—I met Louise and two other Brigham[19] faculty, Joia Mukherjee and David Walton, emerging from that makeshift hospital under a tent. Even there, close to the wide-open space of the airport, the charnel-house stench was everywhere. Louise had not slept in days and was signing out patients and duties to her Haitian and American colleagues so that she could rest and come back. Others, bringing supplies, were coming in. Before long, she was headed back to Haiti with a planeload of volunteers. En route back, she noted, more than once, "I didn't sign up for earthquakes."

None of us did. None of us has been trained for such a shock to the body politic; none of us were prepared to manage such destruction and need. Other self-described experts informed us gravely that they *were* so prepared, but privately, at least, we remain unconvinced. We are in uncharted territory here, and a certain humility about diagnoses, prescription, and prognosis is surely warranted.

So what *is* to be done? In clinical medicine, there is a logic to the evaluation of every patient and, as physicians working in Haiti, we quite naturally used this logic every day, not only as physicians caring for individual patients but also when contemplating the enormity of the problems facing a country we care for deeply. What, we kept thinking, was the correct diagnoses, the best treatment plan, and the most realistic prognosis? Because Haiti has long faced social and economic problems, with immense medical and public health challenges rooted in these problems, the earthquake was and is in every sense an "acute-on-chronic" problem. Might addressing the acute needs of the displaced and injured afford us a chance to address the underlying condition?

I.

To answer these questions, we need to know the history of the present illness. There is not time to review that today, so I will use shorthand. Haiti, over two centuries independent, presents with the worst health indices of the Western Hemisphere. Whether we look at malnutrition, maternal mortality, or life expectancy at birth, Haiti is something of an outlier in the region, even if by "region" we mean the United States and Canada *or* Jamaica and Cuba and the Dominican Republic. The question of why this is so, how to explain Haiti's history of growing vulnerability to natural disasters, looms large in any discussion of "building back better."[20]

Today I want to share a few anecdotes that address the role of Harvard Medical School in responding to the crisis in Haiti. I've recounted Louise Ivers's experience and note that the great majority of our colleagues were in Haiti on January 12 because almost all of them are Haitian. But many volunteers began to arrive soon after the earthquake, and we initially focused on bringing in surgical teams. After arriving in the pitch black with a small team of surgeons, anesthesiologists, and an internist, I went to Haiti's largest teaching hospital. One wishes it were the equivalent of, say, the Brigham. But the hospital, dilapidated and underfunded before the earthquake, was understaffed that night and not a single operating room was running. Inside the hospital, there were many bodies and many dying and everywhere the same stench that pervaded the entire city.

There were of course too few personnel and too few supplies. But the director of the hospital was there, as was the chief of nursing—even though it was ten at night and they did not have the tools of our trade. I had last seen them both exactly a month previously, when we had launched a project to feed some of the patients. If there was not enough food for inpatients in Haiti's largest hospital a month prior to the earthquake, imagine what it was like after.

That said, when I returned with President Clinton a week later—he brought surgical supplies and generators and anesthesia, as we'd asked—there were a dozen operating rooms running. In the middle of the hubbub I was proud to see not only teams from the Brigham, Children's, and MGH, but also our own former students and trainees who were managing, along with thousands of Haitian colleagues, an acute-on-chronic affliction evident, at last, to the entire world.[21] An already-bad problem rendered immeasurably worse by the worst natural disaster to befall this part of the world in two centuries.

It's the same thing no matter what health problem you look at. All the cases of tetanus we're now seeing are a reminder of chronic failure to inoculate with an effective safe vaccine that costs pennies. Two nights ago Natasha Archer, a Brigham resident and herself a Haitian-American, wrote to us about the life-saving interventions of a makeshift surgical team from Boston, New York, and New Jersey. A young patient presented with a rigid abdomen late in the evening, had an upright film revealing free air, and was taken to the OR. The diagnosis was ilial perforation, likely from typhoid. She warned, correctly, that a lack of proper sanitation in the coming days and weeks and months would lead to more such cases. I thought, with some shame, that a decade before, I had reviewed the scant literature on typhoid in Haiti, which revealed the same high burden of disease and the same conclusion. A few years before the earthquake, Haiti was declared the most "water-insecure" country in this hemisphere.[22] Again, an acute-on-chronic problem, and one we might finally have a chance to address.

II.

What about the physical exam? That, as we always say in medicine, you have to do for yourself. To palpate and percuss and listen to the patient. Short of that, you have seen the press images of a capital city without a single major federal building left standing. Stop and think what that would look like in this country. But not everyone is equally afflicted, of course, and here is another argument for a more robust approach to global health. An event of this sort is a great leveler in some senses. But this leveling doesn't last long, since those who had food and water and other necessities of daily life before the quake are able to find them more readily after it. A thorough examination of the patient, whether we call it a "post-disaster needs assessment" or something else, must proceed rapidly.

Data are hard to come by—at least hard data. Some say 300,000 dead; others say half of that.[23] One thing is certain: many more will face untimely deaths if the delivery problems we are discussing today are not addressed. Here is what we know 29 days after the quake: a third of Haiti's population of nine million has been affected directly, which means that all Haitians will be affected as the displaced seek safer places to live. An estimated 25,000 government and office buildings have collapsed and, worse, 225,000 homes. This is the reason, along with the inability of the local, national, and international authorities to move swiftly on shelter, that crammed and unsanitary informal settlements have blossomed across the city and to the south; they are spreading north as people seek safe shelter. Haiti, already food-insecure, will have to feed an estimated two million people with a mix of locally grown and imported food. Rainy season is upon us in April and May, and so too is hurricane season.

But it is important not to spurn another kind of data, the qualitative kind: the losses we have all felt. On our Partners In Health team, we mourn friends, colleagues, and family members. None of us will forget Dr. Mario Pagenel, who was so committed to having our work include academic presentations. On the afternoon of the earthquake, he had returned home to work on a presentation, and though we have no proof of death, we have not, and I'm quite sure will not, see him again, since his house collapsed around him. The losses of Dr. Dossous, an intern in St. Marc, and Roodeline Dorcin, a social service intern at Cerca la Source, are representative of the loss of a whole cadre of care providers in training, a loss that will resonate for years and that must be answered with transnational training programs and a coordinated effort to rebuild Haiti's medical training system.

So many others remain unaccounted for.

Not all of our friends lost were Haitian: seven of eight of the U.N. leaders we worked with over the past year perished on January 12. Walt Ratterman, a visionary proponent of solar energy who had worked with PIH in Rwanda, Lesotho, Burundi, and Haiti was in a meeting in Port-au-Prince and has never been found. It was hard to write to his son yesterday, knowing that Walt had gone to Haiti to help us solarize yet another hospital.

One of our senior medical students, Thierry Pauyo, told me during his first year that his dream was to go and work as a surgeon in Haiti, his parents' country but a place he did not yet know. He got his wish and for the past several months has been living in Cange and working with our colleagues to improve surgical care. During the weekends, he stayed with his aunt and uncle in Port-au-Prince, finally getting to know his relatives there. On January 12, his cousins, all eight of them, became orphans. He brought the children to Cange, where they stayed until he could provide safe passage to Montreal: there his parents have taken them into their home. He would be here today, in this auditorium he knows well, if not for a memorial service for his relatives who perished. Such was his first extended taste of his homeland.

On and on the list goes, and it could lead us to forget that the Haitian people are astoundingly resilient in the face of tribulation. A few nights ago, I was leaving a hospital in central Haiti when an old man came up to me and embraced me. "Haiti is finished," he said. I looked to two younger Haitians, a doctor whose family home in Petit-Goave is rubble, and a former patient, now a nursing student, whose school collapsed. "Is it so?"

"No," they both said. "Haiti will never be finished."

III.

What, then, is the diagnosis, that single line that so often follows a long work-up and precedes the treatment plan? My Haitian colleagues insist that recovery is possible, and all those gathered here surely wish to agree with them: this is not a terminal illness. I led with the diagnosis of an acute-on-chronic problem. We saw an enormous earthquake, the acute event, rattle and level the most populated part of the most densely populated country in this part of the world. But "densely populated" is not the chronic part of the equation: poverty is. So the diagnosis is *natural disaster in a setting of great and longstanding privation.*

Haiti needs to be built back much better. This, then, should be the treatment plan, and it is still being formulated and argued over. Infectious disease consultants close their consults with recommendations rather than prescribed plans, as it is the job of the patients' primary providers to decide on and implement those plans. Again, this is helpful logic in contemplating what now lies before us. There are simply too many prescriptions for Haiti. Some are completely discrepant and most do not do enough to strengthen the hand of the Haitian people, who are strong and resourceful and already working to rebuild. How often in medicine have we learned that plans for patients must be, in truth, plans made with patients? How many times have we learned that the image of the doctor working alone is a romantic ideal from another era, that what we need are teams and systems to deliver services effectively? Improving the quality of health care services being delivered—or, as in the current setting, not being delivered—to a courageous people in great need remains our challenge.

Another challenge is resettlement, even as cities and towns are rebuilt. So far, the Haitians seem to be doing this on their own, without much help—or without anything close to as much as they need. Since perhaps the biggest challenge of all is massive job creation, it's notable that some agencies are finally implementing "cash-for-work"—a term we should be embarrassed to use—programs. There were, as of Friday, about 35,000 of these. But what is needed is more on the order of 500,000 jobs just in the next few months, prior to the rainy season. This is the only way to move resources from the self-described donor nations to the victims who are able-bodied and anxious to work.

Schools need to be rebuilt. Prior to the quake, demographers and aid agencies spoke of the "youth tsunami" about to wash over Haiti, speaking at times as if Haitian youth are more of a threat than an asset. But human capital is Haiti's chief asset, and getting children and young people back into schools that are safe and offer modern pedagogy must be a high priority.

And what might be done to help students like those here today? Right after the quake at the general hospital I ran into three young medical students. Their chief concern: "How are we to continue our studies?" Here is yet another role for American universities: to make sure that the current generation of trainees—in medicine and dentistry, nursing, pharmacy, and all of the allied health professions—have a chance to complete their training and serve those in greatest need in Haiti. I recall that Harvard and other universities took in students from Tulane, Dillard, Xavier, and the University of New Orleans after Katrina, and we need to make sure that we have the flexibility to help students from Haiti, too. Yesterday I spoke with my friend and colleague Jim Yong Kim, the President of Dartmouth, and he announced his willingness to help in this regard. We should do the same here and elsewhere.

These are endeavors that would permit us to do no harm. Let us continue to build the pyramid that links research to teaching and to service. Whether we speak of a Brigham infectious disease doctor helping a Dartmouth nephrologist perform the first dialysis in a town in central Haiti or a Children's Hospital plastic surgeon addressing complex surgical problems in a quake-affected hospital, I note in these examples a purity of purpose for the American research university. Whether I refer to a group of students and faculty coordinating volunteers and planes and helping to transfer patients, or to university-affiliated groups willing to raise money for relief and reconstruction, we agree that universities have much to offer even before we get to the in-kind donations of research and teaching that we can offer. In fact, as for Partners In Health and its Haitian sister organization Zanmi Lasante, the great majority of our volunteers, recently, have come from universities like this one.

IV.

Finally, what about prognosis? So many people struggle for survival every day. The proliferation of aid agencies and non-governmental organizations—Haiti counts more NGOs per capita than any other country except India—hasn't helped much. There has been a widely recognized failure to insist that NGO efforts be coordinated in order to strengthen Haiti's development aspirations. This failure is heightened by the avalanche of generous offers now backed up like blood in an obstructed vessel. But the biggest challenge before Haiti is not the lack of coordination of the goodwill efforts. It is that over the years our country and others have failed to support the Haitian people in their efforts to enjoy basic social and economic rights, and now it will be hard to reverse that trend without patience and long-term accompaniment. If I may be permitted one last metaphor, it is impossible to transfuse blood through a 24-gauge needle. Or to drink from a fire hose.

To open up this logjam, we will need to learn, as my colleagues have, how to *accompany* our partners with more than largesse and expertise. We will need solidarity. I've offered you some examples from HMS and from our Haitian partners. There have been other stirring examples. We recently received a message that our rural Rwandan colleagues were dedicating 10 percent of their paychecks to their PIH colleagues in Haiti, and I've counted three fundraisers for Haiti in the city of Kigali. Colleagues in Lesotho raised $20,000 over the past two weeks. So many groups from Harvard have responded. In the PIH office across the river, staff and volunteers—many of them from Harvard and the Brigham—have learned new skills literally overnight, coalescing into extraordinarily effective teams of logisticians and visa expediters and flight coordinators. We are proud and grateful.

V.

I'd like to close by continuing a story I started above. Thierry Pauyo, who I mentioned earlier, recently sent me a picture of himself surrounded by eight now-orphaned cousins. It was labeled "Pauyo plus Eight," which I'm told is a reference to some television show with which I am not yet familiar. For two weeks, this young medical student had to become, up in central Haiti, a sudden parent, much more than a cousin. His chief concern when I saw him ten days ago was to get his cousins to his parents in Montreal.

But Thierry's chief concern, now that they are there, is to return as soon as possible to Haiti, to get back in the operating room, to get back to work. I am inspired by this sentiment, which I feel seeping out of this auditorium. We are anxious to feel it.

For without solidarity—the noblest of human sentiments—much that is good will be washed away. A research university like this one, especially when linked to "effector arms" such as Partners In Health and the Brigham and Children's and MGH, can offer its own brand of pragmatic solidarity that could set the highest standards for scholarship, teaching, and service.

Thank you for what you have done and what you will do in the coming years.

The Tetanus Speech

University of Miami Miller School of Medicine,
Commencement

MAY 15, 2010

Congratulations, fellow doctors! It's an honor to be back among you and a pleasure. Let me start by thanking not only your teachers and the Miller School's leaders, but also by doing the Miami thing and thanking your families for their sacrifices and support. It's close enough to Mother's Day that we should offer a round of applause for all the mothers here today.

But this speech is not for faculty or families. I'd like to send you on your way with counsel that might prove useful over the next few years. Most of you will spend those years in the "see one, do one, teach one" mode. You will be your patients' primary providers, if we count the hours you spend providing, orchestrating, and documenting care. Most of you will be hospital based, although there are more patients and potential patients outside than inside hospitals. So you will be getting only a small part of the picture, if the picture that concerns us as a profession is how we can prevent or relieve human suffering caused by disease.

This may well be the central tension of your lives: how to provide care to the patient in front of you, knowing that so many of the forces that push us all to patienthood are outside of your control.

Will this be a creative tension or a frustrating one? The answer to this question is more subject to your control. Some of you will seek to lessen it by drilling down on a single disease; others will divide time between clinical work and research; still others will look to policy solutions to vexing problems of health care delivery. Each of these strategies is valid, and that's a message I would beg you to take with you as you seek your path forward. Choose a path that will give you satisfaction for at least a couple of decades and be open to striking out in new directions when that satisfaction is diminished. There's a vast world of possibility before you, armed with this degree.

But I know from experience that you're unlikely to remember that I gave you that advice. This is the second graduation speech I've given at the medical school, and there were a few mishaps last time. Although I was trying to show off a bit for various colleagues on the stage, after the speech I learned that those on the platform, due to a fluke in the sound system, didn't hear a word I said.

Further indignities ensued. I sought to measure the efficacy of my speech, hiring a team of consultants to conduct a follow-up survey of each graduate. I went through seventeen IRBs prior to getting the green light to start the study.[24] Our team discovered that only 1.67 percent of respondents remembered anything I said, while 34 percent did not even recall who had given their commencement address. This is both statistically significant and discouraging for a speaker who'd spent hours crafting a long and (I thought) witty speech.

So how does one offer counsel that *will* be remembered? One approach is brevity, and yesterday, at the college commencement, I reminded graduates that Lincoln's most famous speech was only 273 words long. But a non-scientific survey of commencement speeches—a real one—suggests that what people remember are stories. So I am going to tell you three tetanus stories. Two are from Haiti and one from Miami. And I would ask that you always remember that on your first day as fully accredited physicians you heard, from me, The Tetanus Speech.

I.

Story one. Cut to central Haiti, circa 1985. I was at the time splitting my time between Harvard Medical School, where I was a second year student, and central Haiti, where I was working with a small group of Haitian friends to introduce basic health care and educational services to a group of people who had been displaced by a hydroelectric dam and who lived in what must be described as abject poverty. I was full of optimism, in part because I was a young Floridian who had never known abject poverty and did not yet understand the ways in which large-scale social forces constrict possibility. But I was learning a lot about the big picture.

Just as I had never seen abject poverty—"the everyday struggle for food and wood and water," as one Haitian mother described it to me—so too had I never seen tetanus, an exotoxin-mediated systemic disease caused by inoculation of *Clostridium tetani*, an anaerobe for which an effective vaccine was developed in 1924. Remember that date. Growing up, I'd heard of "lockjaw," a classic symptom of tetanus, which causes painful muscle spasms and worse, but cases in the United States were rare, since vaccination is compulsory for public school attendance. In other words, the big-picture story was that sound policies were implemented; the little-picture story, what we see in the hospitals, was almost no disease.

That's not true in the world, of course. Even now, estimates of the total number of cases of tetanus exceed 700,000 per year. I didn't know this number in 1983 and 1984, when I got involved in vaccination campaigns in rural Haiti. If we'd done our job right, I wouldn't have seen any tetanus in that country, since the vaccine is effective and costs pennies. If we'd done our job right, I wouldn't be able to tell you about Josiane.

By 1985, we'd built a small and overcrowded clinic in Cange. I worked mostly with a small group of community health workers, trudging around the countryside doing a health census and meeting with village councils willing to help us expand our prevention programs. One day, a group of men carried a teenage girl into our crowded clinic on a makeshift stretcher. She was wracked with spasms, which all of us recognized instantly as tetanus. In severe tetanus, these spasms can cause a horrible contraction of the paraspinal muscles called opisthotonos, which can even fracture vertebral bodies. That's how Josiane, conscious and suffering terribly, presented.

We didn't know what do to. That is, we knew to look for a wound and debride it and to ease the spasms with muscle relaxants such as diazepam; we knew that antibiotics would likely help and had them on hand. But we also knew that proper care of a patient with severe tetanus requires mechanical ventilation, sometimes for weeks, and we neither had it nor knew where to seek it, even in the capital city.

We dropped a nasogastric tube and began therapy in a quiet and dark room that we dubbed, anxiously, "the ICU." We sent someone to Port-au-Prince to look into possibilities for transfer, although after a couple of years in Haiti I'd become doubtful about the efficacy of such transfers, since so many led to nothing more than a false sense of security. And Josiane began to respond to therapy, with a diminution in the ferocity of spasms; within a couple of days she was able to say a few words without triggering another wave of them, and I began to think our little ICU, even without a vent, might save her life. It was a great feeling. The search of assistance in Port-au-Prince turned up nothing, as the General Hospital was wracked by its own spasms of disorder and the private hospitals in town did not have ventilatory capacity outside of the ORs.

A few nights later, in the wee hours, someone came to look for me, yelling "*Josiane mouri!*" (Josiane is dead.) I sprang from my bed and ran to her room, asking for others to look for the real doctors. But as I examined the patient, I saw her breathing raggedly. Had we oversedated her? Were her diaphragmatic and intracostal muscles affected? Was it autonomic dysfunction, the cause of many cardiac deaths among patients with severe tetanus? Had we failed her in the little-picture sense, by providing the wrong care, just as we'd failed her in the big-picture sense, by failing to vaccinate? I felt terrible and remember this as an epiphany of dread, one which would become familiar to me as the years ticked by.

But Josiane did not die. She recovered: our distal interventions saved her life. She later married and had a family and, as far as I know, is doing just fine, this quarter of a century later. A happy ending, and there are many of those in medicine, as you will see in your careers.

What this left me with, as a 25-year-old medical student, was a deep respect for the potential power of life-saving, if distal, medical interventions, and I made a private pact with myself to spend my life seeking to bring decent medicine to people living in poverty. That includes building better medical infrastructure and also building human capacity to prevent disease or bad outcomes whenever possible. Now I am lucky enough to work with thousands of Haitian colleagues scattered from the Dominican border to the coast at Saint-Marc who help run a dozen hospitals in rural Haiti.

II.

Story two concerns the earthquake in Haiti. Again, it's a big-picture/small-picture story. Anyone in Haiti, or anyone who has worked in Haiti, can tell you where they were at five in the afternoon on January 12, when the earthquake struck. Having just left Haiti with my family, I was in this very city. It seems like years ago.

You can imagine the anguish, and I do not wish to darken this celebration by commenting on it overmuch. But imagine trying to practice medicine in the midst of such destruction. As noted in story one, we need the tools of our trade to do a good job. What tools were needed most, and how could we get them?

Some of what was needed was all too clear. As with Josiane, we needed ICU-level care, hard to come by in the days and weeks after the quake. It would take a long time to list all of the contributions of the Miller School to the task at hand. But the one for which I am most grateful was the life-saving care for thousands of injured patients, a few with tetanus but most with crush injuries and every other sort of trauma. Within days, the UM and Medishare put up a large field hospital, a place where all but the worst injuries could be managed; many here helped us to transfer, to Miami and elsewhere, those who could not be helped in Haiti. Over 300 UM faculty and senior trainees, from surgeons to nurses, flew to Haiti to save lives. Please join me in thanking UM's health professionals for countless acts of pragmatic solidarity.

But we're far from where we need to be. Because Haiti's is an acute-on-chronic problem, there will be many more health complications of the quake and subsequent displacement of over a million people. In fact, there will be many more tetanus cases unless we link the big picture to the small one. Tomorrow I am headed to Penn, where I will see another tetanus patient on whom I've been consulting informally. Who knows what portal of entry was afforded to clostridia in this perilous time after the quake? His name is Ricot, and he's been vented now for a couple of weeks, his course complicated by the autonomic dysfunction. We think he'll make it, but it's unlikely he would have if he'd remained in Haiti, where ICU beds remain in short supply.

III.

The third and final tetanus story takes place in the United States and allows me to end on a lighter note. Some of you know that my youngest brother, Jeff, works at Miller. He started working with the dean a few years ago, as the Director of Fitness—this following a storied career as a professional wrestler. For those of you who cannot see my bulky sibling, who is sitting right in front of me, let's just say that we don't look too much alike. My tenure in wrestling, or any other sport, was short lived; I never had to face that tough choice between pro football and World Championship Wrestling. When we first traveled together in Haiti, an old man looked at us and asked, simply enough, "Same mother, same father?"

How, you're thinking, will I get a third tetanus story into The

Tetanus Speech? A month ago, my brother stepped on a nail in Coconut Grove. So I said, as you might expect, "get a tetanus booster." Then I sent him a barrage of email reminders, since I have seen so much tetanus that I am haunted by the unlikely but bad cases that occur too often in my line of work. We both knew he'd had tetanus vaccine before, but when? It seemed obvious that there was no downside to playing it safe.

After some fraternal-avuncular pestering, Jeff started calling the obvious places. On the first call he was asked who his primary care provider was. My brother unwisely told the truth: "I don't have one." Then you have to have one, they told the erstwhile and hulking Director of Fitness for the Miller School. Then my brother did the smart thing and made something up: "Lanny Gardner is my PCP."

"Please hold."

The next thing you know, my brother is transferred to someplace in Kendall. "But I work right here on the campus of the medical school," he objected mildly.

"Please hold."

Then my brother was transferred to Bascom-Palmer.[25]

"But I don't have tetanus of the eye," he said. "Can you even get tetanus of the eye?"

I insisted, from Haiti and by email, that he try again. By this time he was finding it amusing, one of my brother's great charms but not necessarily helpful in tetanus-prevention activities. He dialed another number.

"Please hold." He held.

Eventually, an even more avuncular voice came on the phone. "Hello?"

"Lanny?" asked my brother.

Now I think all of us agree that you shouldn't need the former chief of medicine to get involved in procuring a tetanus booster. Many of us would argue that it's a process that shouldn't involve physicians at all.

My brother insists I add that once he was in close proximity to the vaccine he received it speedily and fairly painlessly. I reassured him that the dysfunction he described is typical of even the best American medicine: the delivery gap remains our biggest challenge.

IV.

This, then, concludes "The Tetanus Speech." It was far longer than the Gettysburg Address but shorter than the last commencement speech I gave at the med school. My aspiration is inspiration: you will have, throughout your careers as physicians, tools at your disposal that could not have been imagined mere decades before. You will be called to share the fruits of scientific research and your own training with your patients, knowing that we have a long way to go if a vaccine that will soon be a century old cannot be easily obtained for all those who, by virtue of their humanity, need it.

Your generation of physicians faces a great challenge, one that you will have to tackle no matter where you stand on the arcane and, too often, acrimonious debates about health care reform. We have the technology and we have a lot of know-how. We have a vast engine of research capacity that will answer many questions now before us. But we don't yet have a delivery system that we can rely on if we want to attend, collectively, to our patients and potential patients. This is true whether you work in Miami or central Haiti or any other part of the world.

This dilemma is inescapable, but remember my opening

salvo. Seek a path that will bring you personal satisfaction. It is a great thing to be a physician in the twenty-first century and could be greater still. Since this year I am not only a speaker, but a fellow member of the Class of 2010, I close by expressing my gratitude for your support over the years. It means more to me than I can say here today.

Thank you all and good luck.

PART III

Health, Human Rights, and Unnatural Disasters

One common thread in this section, and in the book as a whole, is an argument against the notion that disparities of risk and outcome are random. Such disparities are no more random than are differing impacts of storms that have buffeted Haiti more than its neighbors Cuba and the Dominican Republic and Jamaica—or that of Hurricane Katrina on inhabitants of New Orleans, stratified by income and place of residence. They are, rather, reflections of broader social forces and social structures in which we all participate, whether we are aware of it or not.

Unnatural disasters, including those just mentioned and also runaway epidemics, are a focus of Part III. In exploring this topic, the speeches that follow draw on three complementary paradigms that are often used in global health. These were introduced briefly in the perhaps overly long Skoll speech in Part I, but deserve further mention here.

One, the development paradigm, is fundamentally an argument for progress through investments in health: in order to break the cycle of poverty and disease that prevents the poor from living long and productive lives, we must invest significant resources in health care and education. If, for example, malaria saps the lives of hundreds of millions on a single continent, then economic growth will be slowed until we do a better job preventing malaria and treating those who are sick from it.

A second paradigm, public goods for public health, argues that any communicable disease, including malaria, demands investments in public health designed to prevent transmission. If the disease is airborne, as is true of tuberculosis or avian influenza, this case is strengthened further.

A third relies on notions of human rights. These arguments are intuitively appealing but often encounter skepticism from experts. Merely trying to define a right to health raises knotty questions. But the effort must be made, because rights-based arguments for global health are the most expansive of the three paradigms. A disease that shortens life spans but does not affect economic growth would not merit attention in the development paradigm; non-contagious diseases matter less in the public goods paradigm. Yet remedying all diseases that afflict humankind is the chief goal of global health.

Further, an unrestricted rights-based paradigm addresses the health of the poorest, who are by definition shut out by the commodification of health services—as no other paradigm does. Whenever patients become "clients" or "customers," a situation in which basic advances in medicine and public health are available only to a few—and least of all to those in greatest need—becomes a bit more normal and acceptable. The notion of a *right* to health stands in opposition to the commodification of care.

The following four talks explore these issues in some depth. The first was delivered at the Harvard School of Public Health in 2004, one year into a war waged on the pretext of weapons of mass destruction that in fact did not exist. But while imaginary weapons could unleash the technological fury—the "smart bombs"—of the most advanced countries, it proved harder to muster *weapons of mass salvation* (vaccines, diagnostics, drugs), the pride and promise of scientific and technological progress.

The weapons-of-mass-salvation speech argues that the growth of modern public health, starting in the latter half of the nineteenth century, occurred in large part because technological progress was linked to efforts to advance equity. This link was made most eloquently by Rudolph Virchow, who declared in 1848 that "physicians are the natural attorneys of the poor."[1] Virchow's shadow should loom large over medicine and public health. But other paradigms, including the most noxious one— the commodification of medicine and even public health—have captured the policy base, even if the moral high ground remains firmly in line with Virchow's vision. To make public health matter, we need to remember that rapid advances in medicine and technology must be tied to an equity plan if we are to imagine a future with fewer stupid, premature deaths.

Nothing made the case for equity better than Hurricane Katrina. The Tulane Medical School Class of 2008 began their studies in New Orleans not long after the already forgotten Tropical Storm Jeanne claimed two thousand lives in and around Gonaïves, Haiti. During those students' first month in New Orleans, I had the chance to speak at Tulane and at Charity Hospital. As I headed back to central Africa, Katrina had taken shape in the Caribbean and churned slowly northward through the Gulf of Mexico. By the time I reached rural Rwanda, my colleagues there were already watching, on computer screens and other technologies that could not have been imagined a decade previously, the grievous landfall of New Orleans's storm of the century. Tulane, like other institutions there, closed and sent its students elsewhere for months; even Charity Hospital, founded in 1736, faltered.

Unlike Tropical Storm Jeanne, which strafed Haiti and its neighbors, Hurricane Katrina would live on in memory as a reminder of the fallibility of not only public health but of all institutions charged with public safety and disaster preparedness. The importance of race and class and all of the large-scale social forces mentioned in the previous sections of this book were laid bare for all to see. Even to observers in rural Rwanda, the social fault lines of a wealthy and technologically advanced society were in clear and scandalous view.

Unnatural disasters were very much on my mind even then, a year before Haiti was rocked by four such storms in a single month (putting Gonaïves under water once again), and two years before an earthquake laid waste to Port-au-Prince.

Of all disasters other than war and famine (which often come as a pair), earthquakes are the most deadly. They have the highest immediate mortality rates; most die within hours of the initial event. The Richter scale quantifies the shaking of the earth but does not tell us about the number of lives lost and buildings destroyed. What makes for variability in loss of life?

A 7.3 quake in another country or city would have had an entirely different aftermath. A more powerful earthquake in Chile on February 27, 2010, claimed fewer than 600 lives, compared to the hundreds of thousands lost not two months prior in Haiti. The poor quality of Haitian construction, the city's tenuous perch on a steep mountain, the overcrowding, the lack of preparation or rescue equipment and personnel, the long-term divestment from public institutions that should have led the response, and the extreme political disarray that had led to the presence of foreign peacekeepers from as far away as South Asia—all conspired to amplify the impact of the Haitian quake and to worsen its after-effects. The cholera epidemic that followed had several causes, the absence of clean water and the presence of peacekeepers from cholera-endemic regions chief among them. That the cholera strain was a new pathogen in Haiti underlined the social determinants of epidemic disease and pointed to connections between countries at opposite ends of the world.

Building a broader sense of the commons—beyond nationality—will guarantee our entire species a share of the fruits of scientific progress, regardless of where we happen to be born or to fall ill.

But alongside new scourges, such connections can bring salves—weapons of mass salvation, even.

Global Health Equity and the Missing Weapons of Mass Salvation

Harvard School of Public Health, Commencement

JUNE 10, 2004

It's a great honor to address you today. I was in Haiti in April when it was announced that I'd be speaking today, and I received an email from one of my HSPH students. He wrote, "I heard you're the commencement speaker this year . . . you beat out Bono!" He's here today—the student, not the singer—and I plan to ask him what he meant. I admire Bono a great deal—he's a fine singer, fills stadiums—and decided to take it as a compliment. It reminded me that Bono once opened a Harvard commencement address by noting, "I'm really nervous. I've never spoken in front of a crowd this small before."

I'm nervous, too, because this is my first commencement speech at a school of public health. It's more challenging than a med school address. There are annoying, general rules: partisan politics are to be avoided. If mention of war is made, it should be to wars conducted in previous centuries and made into films starring Brad Pitt. Then there are the special public health house rules. One needs, always, to use the terms "prevalence" and "incidence." Also encouraged are "population-based" and "burden of disease." Biostats are not required for events like this, but good public health jokes and anecdotes are.

This is a problem. How many of you know any public health jokes? Ours is not what I'd call a hilarious field. Worse, jokes must have broad cultural salience since the average HSPH class usually has students from 64 countries, speaking, collectively, more than 147 languages, not counting the public-health-speak in which you are now fluent.

Here's a cross-cultural public health joke, which I first heard in the cafeteria next door. The Declaration of Alma Ata, signed by World Health Organization member states in 1978, is considered a milestone in the contemporary primary health care movement. The goals were lofty—"health for all by the year 2000"—but the plans that were put forth, from improving vaccination coverage to decreasing malnutrition, were deemed feasible by signatories. But these objectives were not met in most of the countries in which such victories were needed most. Some of the poorest countries registered worsening health indices. As the year 2000 approached, the Alma Ata slogan became the butt of ridicule in international health circles. The slogan contained a typo, went the joke: the rallying cry had really been "health care for all by the year *3000*."

You see? Not hearing any belly laughs out there. Public health jokes are pretty much dark humor. Because the stakes are high. When the stakes are high, so too must be our standards. But instead we've seen, in the name of pragmatism, a ratcheting down of expectations when addressing the health of the poor. This has been a major problem: setting low standards for populations living in poverty is now the "default mechanism" in international health. As you begin or resume your careers, you'll have to deal with the conventional wisdom that leads us to set our sights low for the world's bottom billion.

Where should *you* take public health? I'm no historian of the field but have the impression that there have been high and low points in public health. To confirm this impression, I did some original research, the results of which I'll present here. I'll turn later to nineteenth-century public health, but first a word from our sponsor, the twentieth century. Only four years into this one, we're standing on the shoulders, sometimes stooped, of twentieth-century leaders. Those leaders and their colleagues struggling in the vineyards were my research subjects. I set out to do research on public health practitioners in the contiguous United States and the U.K. (including the Falklands and Gibraltar).

Most of you have heard of Harvard's famous "Nurses' Health Study" and "Doctors' Health Study."[2] But I'll bet even Barry Bloom didn't know about our "Public Health Practitioners' Study," a population-based survey of 26,000 respondents.[3] We discovered interesting trends and associations. Some are unsurprising: 64.2 percent of those surveyed identified the eradication of smallpox as the crowning achievement of twentieth-century public health. And that was statistically significant, with a p-value of 0.00001.

Our research revealed other interesting associations. First, there is a preponderance of Scorpios and Libras in public health practice, but fully 17 percent of all public health deans in the United States, Scotland, and Wales self-identify as Aries. Second, most public health practitioners believed that cigarette smoking is bad for one's health. Fully 72 percent did not believe that aromatherapy would cure compound fractures; that number rose to 89 percent when respondents from California were excluded from the data set.

These numbers have held steady over the past three decades. During these same years, however, there were changes in international public health. The survey uncovered certain hangdog attitudes and a lot of whining. The refrain was "not enough resources," and research showed that, indeed, little was invested in public health in the 1980s and after, a time of growing global inequality. In an essay titled "A Perfect Crime," the economist James K. Galbraith offers a view of "rising inequality in the age of globalization" by looking at trends during these years. "In the last two decades," he writes in 2002, "inequality has increased throughout the world in a pattern that cuts across the effect of national income changes. During the decades that happen to coincide with the rise of neoliberal ideology, with the breakdown of national sovereignties, and with the end of Keynesian policies in the global debt crisis of the early 1980s, inequality rose worldwide."[4]

Some of you are thinking, "What on earth is neoliberal ideology?" Others, especially those from Latin America and Africa, are nodding knowingly. It's complex, but suffice it to say that neoliberal approaches to public health and medicine involve the commodification and privatization of our services so that they become "products" to be purchased by "consumers." Patients become "clients" or even "customers." Public service becomes private enterprise—that's the neoliberal dream. I don't know if the commodification of public health is bad for everyone, but I know from long years in Haiti that it's bad for those who have no purchasing power: the poor. Those with no purchasing power tend to be the very same souls who bear the greatest burden of disease.

Not all the news is bad. During the same time that Galbraith discerns "the rise of neoliberal ideology," we've seen investments in the basic sciences yield amazing new discoveries, discoveries that could be transformed into weapons of mass salvation (WMSs), such as vaccines. But even scientific progress threatens to be undone by growing global inequality and a commensurate failure to invest in protecting the health of the poorest. Those with access to the fruits of science live longer, healthier lives, while those without are leading shorter and more painful ones. In parts of the world, AIDS has sped up this process so that all can see how fast and miserably the medical have-nots die. This growing "outcome gap" is related to the growing income gap.

Global health emergencies have local echoes and should serve as clarion calls to action. They're why Harvard started a major new initiative in global health; they're why we've launched a new residency in "global health equity" at the Brigham and Women's Hospital. But inside the small, insular world of international public health, we've witnessed the Balkanization and petty skirmishes that always arise in times of scarcity. As global inequality grew, we international health specialists started retreating into our own little fields and found ourselves bickering over small pots of money. In the United States, you'll remember big fights about building NICUs *versus* investing in prenatal care, as if these were mutually exclusive endeavors.[5] Paul Wise, the pediatrician who taught me the term "outcome gap," has showed with devastating clarity how these debates detract attention from the equitable distribution of good "high-tech" care for Americans living in poverty without helping to increase their access to prenatal care.[6]

The situation is more unsettling in poor countries. In discussing the world's most destitute populations, you'll hear our ilk say things like, "No, we can't focus on mental illness because then we won't pay enough attention to infectious diseases." Or:

"You can't *treat* AIDS in resource-poor settings because then there will be no money left for prevention." I swear I saw an argument in which one expert chastised another for focusing on asthma due to cooking fires when the real problem was tobacco. Talk about nerds at war!

How do these skirmishes play themselves out among the poor?

I. A LITTLE TRIP TO EAST AFRICA

Let me answer by telling you about a recent trip to East Africa. To protect the innocent, I won't mention the country, but the trip included stays in Maasailand and near the shores of Lake Victoria. (That narrows it to two countries.) I was traveling with the director of Partners In Health, a group that seeks to remediate inequalities of access to care. We were visiting several AIDS projects. A small one in Maasailand integrated prevention and care, and delivered basic health services to pastoralists who'd never before received them. We flew from Nairobi to the Chyulu Hills, a spectacularly beautiful part of the world. Mount Kilimanjaro rose like a monument; a lot of large mammals milled about on pale green fields dotted with acacia trees. We were in a tiny plane with a Kenyan pilot. (Wait—I wasn't supposed to mention any countries.) I was in the back seat, and to my right was a pile of generic antiretrovirals (ARVs). We buzzed the grass airfield to dislodge the local fauna, which were busy grazing on said airfield.

I'm embarrassed to tell you that I asked the pilot only one question. I pointed to long-necked ungulates munching on the acacia trees and asked, "Are those giraffes?" The pilot barely deigned to answer—"Yes, doctor, those are giraffes"—and shot me a look that said, "No, bwana, they're French poodles." I was too amazed to be embarrassed for long.

The next day we visited patients in clinic and in their homes. The Maasai, as you know, tend to be tall and lean. Several, I noted, were missing a lower incisor, a dark gap right in the middle of their smiles. I asked a friend who'd been working there why. It's removed prophylactically, she said, so that when people get trismus from tetanus—"lockjaw," as it's aptly enough termed—their kin can feed them milk to increase chances of survival.

Now some may think of this as a clever, even charming adaptation to "local conditions." In the odd event that someone living near a hospital falls sick with tetanus, the mere spasms of which can fracture the spine, we put in a nasogastric tube and administer medications and food through it. I suppose a gap in a clenched jaw would be more or less the same idea.

But was it really clever or charming in the last century, much less in our own? The groundwork for the tetanus vaccine was laid in the late *nineteenth* century, for heaven's sake. Looking at the winsome Maasai, I sort of wanted to scream, "WHY NOT VACCINATE THEM INSTEAD OF PULLING THEIR TEETH OUT?" But since the project we were visiting was doing everything from vaccination to integrated AIDS prevention and care, I gave instead a silent prayer of thanks that our hosts were addressing the outcome gap in an effective manner.

The trip to Lake Victoria was more disturbing. There, at ground zero of the AIDS epidemic, where the prevalence of HIV in some communities exceeds 30 percent of the young adult population, we saw a lot of kids and a lot of older people, but not a lot of young adults. Look around you at this graduating class: it was people your age who were missing. A missing generation. Imagine that.

We'd gone there to evaluate programs for orphans and also "home-based care" projects for people living with AIDS. But since the home-based care did not include ARVs, most of the people receiving this care did not survive for long. Our African colleagues running the programs were pretty discouraged. Give us the right tools, they said, and we can make it work.

Certainly, that's been our experience in Haiti. We're often asked why we have so few AIDS orphans in central Haiti, and part of the reason is that, in our neck of the woods, young mothers with advanced AIDS can reasonably hope to receive the same standard of care available here in Boston. Why weren't antiretroviral medications being used more widely on the shores of Lake Victoria? It was clear that AIDS-affected *families* there could not buy even generic ARVs, but what about the transnational *institutions* funding the projects we'd visited? They could afford to integrate HIV prevention and care but had not because they'd been told by experts that it was not "cost-effective" to do so. Not cost-effective, not sustainable, not a ranking public health priority. Imagine hearing this on the shores of Lake Victoria, with its child-headed households, crowded orphanages, and untilled fields. But then again, it's not in such places that these claims are staked, but rather in Boston or Geneva or Washington or London or New York. I have yet to meet a poor person, in Haiti or Africa or around the corner from here, who says, "Don't bother, doc: I don't think care for me is going to prove cost-effective."

This reminds me of another story about AIDS. I was at a conference last August arguing that AIDS prevention and care can reinforce one another. I gave the presentation with a friend, a non-fiction writer who knows a lot about international health. Both of us referred to patients who'd been brought back from the dead with ARVs. It was hot outside and, like any rational people who'd just finished a public address, we were having a beer. Two gentlemen walked up to us—to compliment us, we thought. And indeed, the opening gambit of one was to say, "Informative talk, very good." We hoisted our steins amiably.

The same gentleman continued. "But aren't you worried about population growth? I mean, by saving these people's lives, aren't you working on the wrong side of the population equation?"

Now I'd heard this sort of thing many times—never in Haiti, mind you, nor in Africa, but rather at conferences and universities in parts of the wealthy world—and so remained calm. But my friend the writer turned an alarming shade of violet. All sorts of formerly minor veins popped on his brow; his neck went magenta. He's a Vietnam vet, and I was worried things might get ugly, so I tried to play peacemaker. "I'm all for worrying about population control," I said, my brow sweating in time with my beer mug. "I just think there are better tools for it than epidemic disease."

The gentlemen nodded, smiled sunnily, and ambled off. It took at least two more beers before the vasculature on my friend's forehead receded and he faded to his normal ruddy pink.

The gentlemen had a point. Neither of them was a public health specialist, but they were interested in the world and saw its biggest problem as overpopulation. A common enough view. But I'll wager that the majority of the planet's *poor* inhabitants see unequal distribution of the world's bounty, and not overpopulation, as a worse problem.

Either way, mix up overcrowding and inequality, stir, add disease, and you've got yourself a cataclysm. Mind you, I'm not thinking of the cataclysmic deep freeze just presented in the summer blockbuster *The Day After Tomorrow*, although there's nothing quite so delicious, and relevant to the inequality question, as the scene in which U.S. refugees are halted at the border of Mexico. The Americans proceed to cut down a chain-link fence on the U.S. side in order to wade across the Rio Grande into Mexico.

A new ice age may arrive one day, but we're in for trouble right now. Think about violence and conflict and their relationship to the growing outcome gap. I read last week that the current U.S. administration has spent $191 billion on wars in the Middle East. During the same years, we've seen health care in this country take a hit in the name of neoliberal ideology: witness 6 million low-income seniors losing Medicare eligibility, and 3.8 million *more* Americans losing their health insurance. The current administration has cut back on its pledge to fight global AIDS and has imposed strictures on how this aid is to be used. These strictures, including an effective preference for programs that privilege abstinence-based HIV prevention, are often informed by ideology and dogma rather than evidence.

Imagine if we had even half of that war chest, the mere bagatelle of $95.5 billion, for weapons of mass salvation. In contrast to certain WMDs, these weapons do exist. They are vaccines and programs of prevention and care; they are decent sanitation and enough to eat. And don't you wonder if attacking the social problems of the bottom billion might be a more effective means of expunging terrorism than some of the current strategies being employed?

One thing on our to-do list, if we want to make the world a more decent and safer place, is to bridge the gap between public health and medicine and between the haves and the have-nots. How will you all do this?

II. REMEMBERING JOHN SNOW

Let's go back to the nineteenth century—the heyday, sadly enough, of public health—and recall the example of John Snow. You know already that in 1854, after investigating a London outbreak of cholera, he sought a meeting with the local health authority called, aptly enough, the Board of Governors and Directors of the Poor. The Board's records show that "Dr. John Snow has respectfully requested an interview with them. He was admitted and presented an account of his investigation so far. As a result the committee issued an order that the handle be removed from the Broad Street pump." The pump handle was removed the next day, and the cholera epidemic subsided.

There's a lot more to Snow than this famous story. As a pioneering anesthesiologist and activist, he fought suffering on several levels. On March 5, 1855, for example, Snow walked to a poor neighborhood to administer chloroform so a "fragile young man" could have teeth extracted. Then onto the Mayfair district, where he chloroformed an old guy having dead bone debrided from his leg—imagine having that done without any anesthesia, as had been standard practice. Then Snow crossed the River Thames to help remove a kidney stone.

That was just the morning. Later that day, Snow testified before the Houses of Parliament. The English were leaders in the process of gentrification and the city's grandees were trying to get rid of what they called "the offensive trades." They weren't talking about the precursors of Enron or Halliburton, but rather "trades that released foul-smelling, noxious fumes," like bone boilers and tallow melters. In Snow's biography, we read that the "sanitary reform movement was driven by the medical opinion that poisonous vapors, whether miasmas rising from marshes or from decomposing organic matter near human dwellings, were the main cause of disease, including epidemic cholera, which had killed tens of thousands of people in England since 1831."[7]

Snow regarded the miasma theory as rubbish, and said as much to the select committee seeking to remove the offensive trades. In a famous book, he presented "two landmark epidemiological studies of cholera that would secure his reputation into the twenty-first century: an analysis of the differential mortality in thirty-two London subdistricts supplied by two companies drawing water from separate stretches of the Thames, and also the linkage of a lethal Golden Square outbreak to contamination of a popular pump at Broad Street."[8]

The select committee was not very friendly to Dr. Snow. Unlike Condoleezza Rice, John Snow couldn't review the questions ahead of time. He noted, "I have paid a great deal of attention to epidemic diseases, more particularly to cholera, and in fact to the public health in general; and I have arrived at the conclusion with regard to what are called offensive trades, that many of them do not assist in the propagation of epidemic diseases, and that in fact they are not injurious to the public health."

Snow was then questioned by one Sir Benjamin Hall. "Are the Committee to understand," Hall inquired incredulously, "taking the case of bone-boilers, that no matter how offensive to the sense of smell the effluvia that comes from the bone-boiling establishments may be, yet you consider that it is not prejudicial in any way to the health of the inhabitants of the district?"

"That is my opinion," Snow replied. The problem, he showed, lay elsewhere.

A contemporary of Snow's, Rudolph Virchow, once argued: "Medicine, as a social science, as the science of human beings, has the obligation to raise . . . problems and to attempt their theoretical solution; the politician, the practical anthropologist, must find the means for their actual solution."[9]

Here you are, gathered together for commencement. Many of you are already seasoned practitioners; some are scientists; others will be ministers of health; still others are just starting. But all of you are dedicated to raising problems and finding solutions. It is my firm belief that the global outcome gap is the biggest problem facing medicine and public health.

III. HEALTH AND HUMAN RIGHTS

Primary health care nerds like us warring over scarce resources, the outcome gap, the gap in Maasai incisors, the missing generation on the shores of Lake Victoria, famous dead white guys who cared little for effluvia—what do these all have in common?

All concern human rights, for starters. Your diploma comes with a copy of the Universal Declaration of Human Rights, which is worth reading often. But, alas, even this noble framework will not lead us out of quagmires like terrorism, Iraq, the proper treatment of prisoners in this country or any other, the need to roll out AIDS treatment in Africa, the need for national health insurance. There is no single compass for so diverse an endeavor as public health as you will practice it across this broad world. You'll be called to ask hard questions about the very real incompatibilities between violence—including wars—and public health. Between unfettered accumulation of wealth and persistent poverty.

Asking these questions might not win you popularity contests. But then everyone knows you're going into public health for the money.

Seriously, public health practitioners are called to stand with the sick and those most likely to become sick. Even those of us who are predominantly clinicians are still called to address the root causes of human suffering, as Virchow and Snow did. I've been accused by my friends of abusing a bit of verse by Bertolt Brecht. It's called "A Worker's Speech to a Doctor."

> When we come to you
> Our rags are torn off us
> And you listen all over our naked body.
> As to the cause of our illness
> One glance at our rags would
> Tell you more. It is the same cause that wears out
> Our bodies and our clothes.
>
> The pain in our shoulder comes
> You say, from the damp; and this is also the reason
> For the stain on the wall of our flat.
> So tell us:
> Where does the damp come from?[10]

Public health is all about telling us where the damp comes from and finding solutions. Allow me to close by underlining three issues that you will have to face in your practice of public health.

The first concerns social justice. We desperately need a new equity plan. The nineteenth-century champions of public health believed that social justice was central to their endeavors. Since then, science has helped us to develop new weapons of mass salvation, but we need an equity plan if we are to get these life-saving interventions to those who need them most.

Second point: we need alternatives to the Balkanization of medicine and public health. AIDS is simply a metaphor for the rest of it. In integrating prevention and care, we make common cause between clinicians and epidemiologists and policymakers and scientists and activists. Between patients and healers. Between rich and poor.

Third point: the fight over "scarce resources" involves no small amount of chicanery. There are enough resources on this planet to do the job right. These resources are far less than those required to wage wars whose justifications are never quite as good as *their* champions make them out to be. When you are bold in pressing for the right to health care rather than arguing how best to spend paltry sums that could never do the job, or even half the job, you advance the cause of public health.

There. I kept my promises, except the one about brevity. I used all the technical terms required. I bowed to giants of public health. I made three points. I talked about current events, including the touchy subjects, but leavened these references with allusions to pop culture. I even told public health jokes.

But if public health itself is not to become a joke, we're going to have to pull together to develop an equity plan that is worthy of both our weapons of mass salvation and the world's great need for them.

You're the generation charged with this task, and all of us here wish you well as you remake the world before it is too late.

Congratulations and thank you all.

Making Public Health Matter

Bloomberg School of Public Health
(Johns Hopkins University), Commencement

MAY 24, 2006

The first thing I'd like to say is hello, public health warriors, and congratulations!

I take graduation speeches seriously and try to do research about my host institution. I like speaking at public health commencements in part because there's no school song and no lacrosse team. But it's still difficult to give a cheerful yet serious speech of great relevance at such a diverse gathering. Your families are here. Your friends. Teachers of biostats as well as policy wonks. People from red states and blue; Muslims, Christians, Jews. Cost-effectiveness gurus and human rights–types. Left brain, right brain. Scorpios and Libras. Vegetarians and carnivores. Doctors and epidemiologists. Venusians and Martians. Mac and PC. Et cetera.

The job, I later learned, is to entertain and instruct, but primarily to entertain. The instruct part I get, and that's why I've titled this talk "Making Public Health Matter." I'd be so honored if you were to remember this theme, which is about an equity plan for medicine and public health, even if you don't remember my name or title or the color of my robes. And the robes are goofy. Half the people here look like they're about to get off the Hogwarts Express.

So one can resort to inside humor regarding the experience you've all just been through here in Baltimore these past few years. You know, local color. But as I thought about it, I know this city far less well than I should. Before I speak about Baltimore, though, let me tell you an instructive little story about a road trip through the Midwest. It reflects a few key themes and will entertain you in large part by its brevity, which is, as commencement speakers soon learn, the key to success.

I.

So the story: a relation of mine was in St. Louis attending a religious gathering, and he was taken ill. He had something of a psychotic break and was taken to a private hospital not far from the city. He was pretty wigged out (to use jargon from the *Diagnostic and Statistical Manual of Mental Disorders,* Volume 7R). It wasn't as if he could fly back to Boston, so I decided to fly out and rent a car to drive him back. There were some insurance issues—as in, he had none—and the clock was ticking. It's not as if the private hospital threatened to kick him out, but the meter *was* running. We wanted to get him back to his regular doctor in Boston.

I conferred with my sister, who lives in Kansas City. We decided I'd fly to KC and then we'd drive to St. Louis, collect our kinsman, and drive him back to Boston. A road trip.

My sisters are all a lot of fun, but this one, sibling number five, is particularly outrageous. She decided she'd rent the car. I'm embarrassed to say this in the middle of an oil war, but my sister decided to rent a roomy car for the long drive to Boston. "Upgrade," she said as she walked out of the rental place jingling the keys to a shiny white Cadillac.

Inside, on the dashboard, it said, "Equipped with On-Star."

I didn't have a clue what On-Star was, but there were many other distractions—papers to sign, bills to worry about. I remember going over the disappointingly small Mississippi River and looking for the Arch. East we tooled, the big Caddy increasing our dependence on Middle East oil with every mile, my sister at the wheel, our patient safely in the back.

All was well until my sister started fiddling with the rearview mirror. She must've accidentally pushed a button because suddenly a mellifluous male voice filled the car: "This is Greg from On-Star. What's your roadside emergency?"

Now this startled me a great deal, but fortunately our kinsman was well medicated. God created trazodone for a reason.

A pregnant pause ensued. Finally, my sister asked, "God, is that you?"

"No, this is Greg from On-Star. How may I help you?"

"Hi Greg," said my sister in what she calls her telephone operator voice. "We didn't mean to trouble you. I was trying to adjust the mirror and inadvertently pressed your button."

"It's no trouble, ma'am," said Greg, voice still booming. "Anything I can do for you?"

Most people would've left it at that, but not my sister.

"Well, Greg, where are you exactly? What are you wearing?"

"We're not authorized to say, ma'am, but should you have trouble we know exactly where you are."

My sister: "What, is this part of the new wiretapping program? Have you wiretapped my Caddy? I thought I swept this thing for bugs."

Greg (sincerely): "No ma'am. It's a GPS unit mounted in the car. We're here to serve."

Sister: "Do you offer a complete range of services? How about universal health insurance? That's what we need today, if you could help us out."

My sister could've kept this up for a long time, I knew, so I intervened in older-brother fashion and searched for the button that would make Greg go away. Finding nothing, I thanked him and let him know that, grateful to be on his grid, we were set for now, thanks. Goodbye.

Even after he signed off, we thought he might still be listening in. You know the feeling, these days? Like they're always listening? But that didn't stop my sister. She was on a roll. "On-Star. Wouldn't it be great," she said, "if whenever you had a crisis of any sort you could just press the On-Star button?" For the next couple of states, at least until Niagara Falls, we went through countless dire scenarios from which we might have wished to be saved. Forty million uninsured? Time to press On-Star! Decreased investments in public health? On-Star! Wait, no vaccine for AIDS, tuberculosis, and malaria, the top three infectious killers in the world today? Press On-Star! Oops—we're at war. Press On-Star. Genocide in Darfur? Hurricane season almost here?

You got it. Press a magic button. But in spite of all the Hogwarts robes around here, there is no magic wand to wave. Making medicine and public health matter for everyone is going to take a lot of work on the part of all of those graduating these days.

OK, so I may have embellished the story. But the part about the hospital was true. The part about renting a big white Cadillac was true, and so was the story of Greg from On-Star. In fact, he's probably listening in right now, especially if you're a Verizon customer.

So how's this story related to equity in medicine? Well, for starters, there's the whole lack-of-insurance thing. A good friend of mine, Howard Hiatt, titled a book about the U.S. health care system *Medical Lifeboat* because he was concerned, as a leader in American medicine, about the leaks sprung in our health care system. In introducing the paperback edition in 1989, Hiatt said he hoped the title was "alarmist enough. The problem certainly is that bad."

I work with Howard Hiatt, and I can tell you that, to this day, he wants to make medicine matter. Here's what he wrote, almost 20 years ago, about our health care system:

> How much worse must it get before we confront it seriously? "Lifeboat?" Passengers don't "take to boats" unless their ship is wrecked or foundering. The American ship of health is not yet on the rocks, at least not for most Americans, but it is headed that way, and in this last year alone it picked up speed.[11]

In the decades since Hiatt wrote his book, the ship has in many respects continued to gain speed.

II.

By now I hope I've sucked you in enough to get to the point. How do we make medicine and public health matter today? You may think I plan to speak about our work in Haiti or Rwanda, and I will. But we have serious problems right here in our bountiful country, as all of you graduating today know already. Is it really worse than what Howard Hiatt described two decades ago? Well, I don't want to be a downer on this day of celebration, but I'll note that our expenditures have risen even further, and not only because we have an aging population. Costs have doubled in a couple of decades, but our health indices have not improved; some have gotten worse. This week, Save the Children reported that, of 33 industrialized countries surveyed by the World Health Organization, the United States is tied for having the second-highest infant mortality rates.[12]

Two weeks ago, on May 5, economist Paul Krugman asked, in the *New York Times*, "Is being an American bad for your health?" He argued that this was indeed the implication of a study just published in the *Journal of the American Medical Association*. After reviewing better-known facts, including the obvious one that we spend more on health care than any other developed nation and yet have worse health indices than Canada, most European nations, and Japan, he turned to the new study, which was titled "Disease and Disadvantage in the United States and in England." Krugman continues his review:

> The authors of the study compared the prevalence of such diseases as diabetes and hypertension in Americans 55 to 64 years old with the prevalence of the same diseases in a comparable group in England. Comparing us with the English isn't a choice designed to highlight American problems: Britain spends only about 40 percent as much per person on health care as the United States, and its health care system is generally considered inferior to those of neighboring countries, especially France. Moreover, England isn't noted either for healthy eating or for a healthy lifestyle.

(As a parenthetical, England isn't known for its dental care, either.)

> Nonetheless, the study concludes that "Americans are much sicker than the English." For example, middle-age Americans are twice as likely to suffer from diabetes as their English counterparts. That's a striking finding in itself.

What's even more striking is that being American seems to damage your health regardless of your race and social class. . . . Americans are so much sicker that the richest third of Americans is in worse health than the poorest third of the English.[13]

Pretty startling stuff to read in May 2006. I know that access to health care is not always the chief determinant of health outcomes. But access is always important. And improving access to our services is in part your job, no?

What happens when we insist on equitable access to care? Take a look at the delivery of AIDS care in Baltimore. Although the variability of AIDS treatment outcomes has been especially obvious in the era of antiretroviral therapy (ART), it was so even before effective therapy became available. Leaving aside disease distribution, some might expect that an untreatable disease would run the same course in all patients once infection occurs. But diagnosing and treating the chief opportunistic infections that were the cause of death among people living with AIDS did not wait on the development of specific antiretroviral therapy and specific serologic tests. In the United States, the ranking opportunistic infection was *Pneumocystis carinii* pneumonia, and delays in diagnosis and initiation of therapy proved fatal to many; so did interruptions in the lifelong suppressive therapies required to control this and other opportunistic infections. In Baltimore in the early 1990s, it was possible to show that race was associated with the timely receipt of therapeutics: among patients infected with HIV, blacks were significantly less likely than whites to have received antiretroviral therapy or PCP prophylaxis when they were first referred to an HIV clinic, regardless of disease stage at the time of presentation.[14] The timeline from HIV infection to death was further shortened in situations where the far more virulent tuberculosis was the leading opportunistic infection, as it is in much of the poor world.[15] The "natural history" of AIDS is a mirage.

This was clear to researchers and clinicians in Baltimore, who described what they termed "excess mortality" among African Americans without insurance. Although such terminology was not used in the studies reviewed here, it is possible to argue that racism and other forms of "structural violence" were embodied as excess mortality. What else accounted for racial disparities in clinical outcomes? Regardless of semantics, few epidemiologists seeking to understand the AIDS epidemic in the United States were able to ignore the social determinants of both distribution and outcome of this disease. Absurd as it may sound, some even argued for intrinsic "racial" susceptibility to poor outcomes.

As epidemiology, the standard "risk factors," which did not consider racism and poverty, did not lead far. But after documenting racial disparities in survival, clinicians and researchers in Baltimore asked what would happen if race and insurance status no longer determined who had access to care, even before treatment routinely included three-drug ART. They didn't press On-Star; they tried to remove barriers to care.

In addition to seeking to remove the obvious economic barriers at the point of care, thought was given to transportation costs and other incentives, as well as comorbid conditions ranging from drug addiction to major mental illness. Improvements in community-based care, conceived to make AIDS care more convenient and socially acceptable for patients, were also implemented. The goal was to make sure that nothing within the medical system or the surrounding community prevented poor and otherwise marginalized patients from receiving the standard of care.

The results registered just a few years later were dramatic:

disparities in outcomes related to race, gender, injection-drug use, and socioeconomic status almost disappeared within the study population.[16] In other words, these program improvements may not have dealt with the lack of national health insurance and still less the persistent problem of racism and urban poverty, but they did lessen the embodiment of social inequalities as premature death from AIDS.

The Baltimore experience has implications for the future course of the U.S. AIDS epidemic; it has implications for all those concerned with poverty and inequality in the United States. The cost of having the cult of the market dictate who has access to what care is bad enough in a rich country, as we've seen. It's devastating in the places in which my colleagues and I work.

In case you can't readily imagine this, I'll give you a vivid example. I was in Rwanda during the month of March. Partners In Health had been asked by the Clinton Foundation and by the Rwandan Ministry of Health to come to rural Rwanda to do three things: to help rebuild the public health sector, to start an integrated AIDS-prevention-and-care program, and to train Rwandans to do work similar to what we've done in Haiti. Just a year ago, we went to the place that would be our new home: Rwinkwavu. What we found was a hospital abandoned since the war and genocide of 1994. In two districts with a population close to 400,000 people, there wasn't a single physician. Not one.

We had our work cut out for us, but we knew what we were doing, even if we couldn't push the On-Star button. The "we" in question included some of our Haitian colleagues, a handful of PIH docs, and a whole lot of Rwandans we recruited and trained. To make a long story short, it worked: within eight months, we reopened the hospital and nearby clinics, enrolled more than a thousand patients on AIDS treatment, and trained over 300 Rwandans to do the work.

I promised vivid examples of the need for a right to health care. On Wednesday, March 22, I was taking morning report. For those of you who are not physicians, "taking morning report" means having a senior physician listen to whatever cases the medical staff might want to present. That morning, I heard about what we call, in the lingo, "pus under pressure." We went over a couple of cases and then went forth into the wards to see some patients. One young boy in the pediatric ward had been on antibiotics for days but still had a fever and was sick because there was a liter of pus in his left thigh.

In this instance there *is* an On-Star button you can push, and it's called a scalpel—you have to drain deep infection if you want to cure it. Some of you hear a metaphor coming, but metaphors are a necessary evil in graduation speeches.

I know that this will seem overly dramatic, but it's nonetheless true that I had seen, by 10 a.m., the following patients: a dozen young people or children affected with AIDS, tuberculosis, or malaria; a young man bitten by a cobra (we gave him, for free of course, antivenin we'd ordered from South Africa); and two boys who were out herding cattle—they'd never been to school, and one was an orphan—and had the misfortune to mistake a landmine for a toy of some sort.

Everyone survived, but it was pretty touch-and-go and required a lot more than just a scalpel and some antibiotics. What do you do when you're poor and get bitten by a cobra? When you're poor and pick up a landmine? There's no On-Star button to press. How do we make medicine and public health matter in rural Rwanda? Not by selling them as commodities. The only way we can use modern medicine in rural Rwanda is to make sure that it's available to all those who need it. Not just to that tiny minority who could pay for it.

We can press On-Star all we want, but Greg's not going to help us with our current health predicament. Our predicament—your predicament—does not concern the future of medical discovery. We don't know where medicine's going, but it's on the right track, as far as discovery goes. Those of us who are clinicians rely on bench science for new diagnostics and therapeutics. And medical science, the youngest science, is moving rapidly and still gathering speed. But here too we need an equity plan: basic science discoveries, even those that would give us vaccines or better drugs for AIDS, will not matter to the destitute sick if we have no plan for distributing them. That's true even in our own wealthy country. I'm afraid we've picked up a delayed-release landmine. Or, to mix metaphors further, we have some pus under pressure in our system and need to drain it before we get gangrene.

This is the primary task of modern public health practice. Do we have the tools? Can we develop them?

III.

Let me close, and answer in the affirmative, by offering a brief tribute to a friend and mentor, J. W. Lee. Dr. Lee was the Director-General of the World Health Organization until he died suddenly this past weekend. In the summer of 2001, when Dr. Lee was heading up WHO's tuberculosis program, he encouraged me to take a larger role in advocacy for increased investment in public health. When he heard that I'd be briefing Congress on the need for more basic science research to develop vaccines for AIDS and tuberculosis and malaria, he gave me a book, Richard Rhodes's *The Making of the Atomic Bomb*, and said, simply, "Read about the copper shortage."

I found the relevant passages. Brigadier General Leslie R. Groves, a leader of the Manhattan Project, wrote that one of his predecessors, Colonel Kenneth Nichols, had been charged with addressing "one serious problem of supply." I quote from Richard Rhodes's book:

> The United States was critically short of copper, the best common metal for winding the coils of electromagnets. For recoverable use the Treasury offered to make silver bullion available in copper's stead. The Manhattan District put the offer to the test, Nichols negotiating the loan with the Treasury Undersecretary Daniel Bell. "At one point in the negotiations," writes Groves, "Nichols . . . said that they would need between five and ten thousand tons of silver." This led to the icy reply: "Colonel, in the Treasury we do not speak of tons of silver; our unit is the Troy ounce." Eventually 395 million troy ounces of silver—13,540 short tons—went off from the West Point Depository to be cast into cylindrical billets. . . . The silver was worth more than $300 million.[17]

I briefed Congress shortly after September 11, 2001, hoping that mine is not an unseemly reference, since what I was pleading for was new *instruments of mass salvation*, rather than weapons of mass destruction. But imagine if the can-do mentality and scientific sophistication that gave us, in short order, a weapon of mass destruction were to be turned to the promotion of global health equity. Imagine a Manhattan Project for the diseases of the poor.

That, dear graduates, is the cause you've taken up. The war against the major infectious killers is also the war against poverty and social inequalities, which are bad enough within our borders and scandalous beyond them. The ways to address social ills are contested bitterly. But we know how to prevent or treat diseases that kill tens of thousands each day. Let us respond with increased investment in the basic sciences, in clinical investigation and new drug development, and in the effective distribution of the fruits of this research to all those who suffer. Let's make public health really matter, unleashing our power in a novel way: reaching out across boundaries of state and ethnicity and language in order to make common cause with those who bear the microbial burdens of poverty. Thus would we strike a major blow against poverty and social inequality, very often the cause of discontent in the modern world.

So that's my message to the Class of 2006. Go out there, across this country and to the four corners of this world, and make public health matter. The most important way to do this is to think about those poorly served by modern medicine and public health today. They are legion, even in this country. Greg of On-Star is not going to fix this; you're going to have to do it yourselves. The good news is that you have so many tools at your disposal, and we can develop many more if we put our minds to it.

Congratulations to all of you. See you in the trenches.

Unnatural Disasters
and the Right to Health Care

Tulane School of Medicine, Commencement

MAY 17, 2008

What a pleasure to be back in this great city. I'm especially grateful that a former teacher of mine is now your dean, since it means all I have to do to have two nice meals in the French Quarter is to deliver your send-off message.[18]

Congratulations, Class of 2008, and welcome to the remarkable, promising, exciting world of medicine. You're adding MD to your names at a wonderful, challenging time. Since you're members of Tulane med school's Class of 2008, you're also veterans of another experience. You were just starting your second year of medical school when Katrina struck.

Knowing what to say about this has been a struggle for me.

When two days ago I left Boston for N'awlins, I was yammering on the cell phone in a cab. I was talking to someone about what might be the best message I might deliver here today. The driver, Rick, is a good friend of mine, and as he helped me get my bags out of the car, he offered the following, unsolicited advice. These were his exact words: "If you want to be really avant-garde, don't mention Katrina at all."

Now this troubled me, since I respect Rick and had already written a good deal of my comments, leading with some reflections on modern medicine that began with a Katrina story. Everyone has a Katrina story, and I had mine. But was it relevant? Was it good enough for Tulane? All the way here, from Boston to NOLA via Newark, I thought about Rick's advice. I knew he had a point. What could be more tiresome than to have a Harvard professor come and expound various theories and comments about Katrina? I thought I'd had a special vantage point, having last been here at Tulane at the end of August 2005 and having met many members of the Class of 2008 who attended my talk here then, but I wasn't sure.

So I sought more advice, again from someone who was good enough to drive me. Yesterday, Kamond fetched me from a nice hotel in the French Quarter—thank you Tulane!—and took me to the med school to meet with students and some faculty interested in global health. Unlike Rick, 100 percent Bostonian, Kamond is 100 percent New Orleans. Born and raised, he said. When I asked for his advice on my speech, he offered it willingly after I told him my Katrina story in brief. "You should go ahead and say something," he said. "It won't be inappropriate at all. Tell these kids that if they can survive Katrina, they can cope with anything they might see as doctors."

So thank you, Kamond, and here goes.

I.

In almost two centuries, this medical school, in whatever incarnation, has been closed only twice: during the Civil War and in 2005. Katrina, surprisingly, has something in common with war: neither are "natural disasters." Not really. Like so many of the diseases you will soon diagnose and treat, they are man-made disasters. Some would say "human-made" rather than man-made, but at this point, wars and incompetent responses to hurricanes and floods, whether here or in Myanmar, are primarily man-made.

I've been shuttling between Harvard and Haiti for 25 years and am headed back to Boston tonight and then to Haiti. But in the summer of 2005, it became my great privilege to try to take our experience in Haiti to Rwanda, which had made remarkable strides emerging from another man-made disaster—the genocide of 1994. It's a long way from Rwanda to NOLA, and some of my coworkers opined that it was just too far to travel for two days. But as I'd made a promise to go to both LSU and Tulane, I was bent on keeping it. Here was my trajectory as I recall it: Kigali, Rwanda, to Nairobi, to DC, to Cincinnati, to Baton Rouge by plane, and then to NOLA by car, with a friend, a Louisiana native, at the wheel. When we drove by some pumping stations in town, he said, and I'll never forget it: "They're a joke. They don't work. One day, this is all going to be under water."

John the prophet, I'll call him. St. John in a world-class, seersucker suit.

So as chance would have it, I was here at Tulane right before a terrible moment in the history of this city and this country. On August 22, 2005, after giving a talk at the medical center and spending the night in the French Quarter, I boarded a plane for Rwanda. The day I arrived at our hospital there, Katrina formed off the coast of the Bahamas. Well before I recovered from my jetlag, Katrina had unleashed her power in my native Florida and then along the Gulf Coast.

Think about how I was following all of this: in rural Rwanda, there's no television reception. But we had put in place Internet connectivity and trained, in the space of a couple of months, dozens of Rwandans how to use computers. Most of them had never held a laptop, much less used one. But they had become, by September 2005, avid users of this technology, which brought news and images to them as if they were watching CNN from Atlanta.

Thus I saw Katrina in large part through the eyes of my Rwandan hosts. Day after day, images from New Orleans pained me and shocked my Rwandan colleagues. "I can't believe that's what the United States is like," was one of the sentiments I heard most often that week. I also had several friends working as doctors here—including one of my closest friends, who was one of those fighting the good fight for charity throughout the crisis. When a mutual friend urged me to help evacuate our doctor-friend, I wrote back that she probably didn't want to leave until the patients were all accounted for.

That's my Katrina story in a nutshell: I watched it unfold from the heart of Africa and worried about close friends I'd just left behind. But the real devastation of Katrina was revealed less by conventional meteorological metrics—category this or category that—and more by our collective failure to attend to the primary needs of our natural constituency: the sick, the poor, the frail, the hungry, the homeless.

II.

Tulane Class of 2008, you have been through difficult times, but they must also be *revelatory* times. You know, better than I, that there are some lessons to be drawn from your experience, whether you are going into anesthesiology, internal medicine, surgery, basic science research, family medicine, pediatrics, or psychiatry.

How best to express this lesson in a single sentence? Here's my attempt: no matter what you choose to do in medicine, you have an obligation to *think about all those who should be beneficiaries of our vocation.* Katrina laid waste to many things. But it also exposed to all the shortcomings of our medical safety net. It reminded us that not all things in this world should be bought and sold as commodities. Some things should be basic rights.

That, in a nutshell, is your generation's fight. How can we fight to promote the right to high-quality health care? As a *right* for everyone?

To do so, we need to tinker with our biomedical culture. Within that culture are countervailing and contradictory notions. At the Harvard hospital where I trained, there was a sort of machismo. You're supposed to be tough. A "strong intern" is one who leaves few tasks for his or her teammates, even if the patients in question need more attention. In the emergency room, a "wall" is someone who reduces the number of admissions—applauded in this machismo view—and a "sieve" is someone who has the weakness to actually admit a patient.

What's wrong with this picture?

At most of our country's teaching hospitals—in my experience, far and away the best in the world—almost no attention is given to community health centers. Home visits by house staff are unheard of. And so we have these islands of excellence surrounded by neighborhoods in which care for chronic diseases is anything but excellent. I believe that's what you call here in New Orleans "isles of denial."

Since Katrina, much has been done to strengthen links between one of this country's oldest medical schools and the communities that surround it. And you, dear Class of 2008, can serve as living links between the hermetically sealed world of the teaching hospital and those outside it who also need your care.

As medical students, a few friends and I started an organization called Partners In Health. Now, more than 20 years later, we are working in ten countries and have thousands of employees, most of them community health workers. But in every project, we ask doctors and nurses to do home visits. Not because the community health workers can't do them alone but rather because we need *living links* between our health care institutions and the communities we serve. We brought this model from Haiti to several poor neighborhoods in Boston, a few miles from the Harvard teaching hospital at which I teach. I got in a bit of trouble for arguing, in promoting the importance of community health workers and home visits, that all we were trying to do was to raise Harvard's level of care up to Haiti levels.

III.

Allow me also to give you some more personal advice. Most of you will begin internships next year; some of you will do research or spend, as I did, a year away from a university medical center before returning to training. But the experience will be the same: one minute you're a med student and the next you have an MD after your name and you have real responsibilities—often enough, life-or-death responsibilities.

It is in these years that you will develop skills but also come to understand just how critical teamwork is. The romantic notion of being The Doctor, alone in seeking to serve The Patient, goes out the door during internship and residency. Cultivate relationships not only with patients and their families but with nurses— try messing with the vent settings without them and see what happens!—and social workers and pharmacists and the people who keep the hospital clean.

Here's my last point: don't be afraid to be real caregivers. Caregiving forces you to deal with the problem of compassion in its original sense. Compassion means "suffering with." Don't be afraid to suffer with your patients. Whether you're a pathology resident or a med-peds resident, don't listen to those who tell you to maintain your distance. Deal with everyone who walks in the door. And keep your door open.

Your class has been, in my view, one of the most important classes in American medicine. You came here with whatever motivations, but as your second year started you had to confront the reality of Katrina. Which was the reality of race and class in our country.

You are the future of medicine, and many of us are betting on your ability to link your elite training to the needs of millions—no, *billions*—in the world today. When we speak of global health, we do so in an inclusive way. Yes, Haiti and Rwanda are part of this network. But isn't Louisiana also on the globe? Isn't the upper ninth on the globe? Wherever you go, remember you live on this same globe, and you have a leading role to play in transforming modern medicine.

Class of 2008, thank you for having me here in 2005, and thank you for bringing me back today.

Congratulations, dear doctors.

Exploring the Adjacent Possible

Georgetown University, Commencement

MAY 21, 2011

Hello, Hoyas! I'm not sure what a Hoya is, but looking out over the crowd I know that I am contemplating a bumper crop of something good.[19] Your kind-looking faces reassure me: as much as I love Georgetown, I accepted this speaking gig only because it was to occur on May 21, 2011. And that meant I wouldn't have to actually give the talk, since they told me that the Rapture was to have occurred today. Seriously, it's my great privilege to join you not at the End of Days, but rather on your last day as college students, to leave you with a message that might be helpful, and most of all to congratulate you.

The helpful-message part is a taller order than I understood when last sitting under a mortarboard—a hat as obscure in origin as is the term "Hoya." The reason it's difficult, beyond the anxiety of speaking in front of a large and diverse crowd of students, parents, and faculty, is that commencements are by definition also endings. They're time for taking stock, for distilling lessons into potent, short form. Anyone who teaches medical school learns quickly that students are looking for a few "take-home messages," and that the preferred number is three. So here are mine for your class.

I.

First: *try not to forget the broader social world around us and the past upon which it's built.* By "social world," I don't mean all that is not the physical world, but rather the world as it is, with all of us—our problems, our triumphs, our connections—in it. This won't be easy, as your lives change rapidly, moving from the general—the liberal arts education you've just completed—to the specific demands of jobs, graduate studies, and families. Worlds often shrink after graduation; perspectives become limited by greater but more narrow responsibilities.

Take as an example any of the basic sciences. The pace of discovery today is such that even the most arcane and specialized branches of science are best illuminated with multiple points of view and by linking close observation of minutiae to ways of seeing that are rooted in the long and broad view that I'm terming "not forgetting."

Some have taken to calling such thinking "fractal," borrowing a metaphor from physics. I turned to *Merriam-Webster's Dictionary* for the definition of fractal: "any of various extremely irregular curves or shapes for which any suitably chosen part is similar in shape to a given larger or smaller part when magnified or reduced to the same size." In other words, things that look wildly different from one perspective but the same from another perspective, another scale.

There's a bit of mystery whenever disparate parts don't appear to add up to the same whole. If this is true in physics, imagine how true it is in the social world, so irregular and fragmented and unequal. The old-school cliché was "Think globally, act locally." But we need to think fractally, at several scales at once, in order to get our arms around the most vexing problems of our day and in order to innovate in all realms. Take the financial crisis, which has already altered your future: it doesn't take a degree in economics to guess that a certain brand of reductionist, quant-driven thinking made it possible for trading overvalued securitized debt products and reckless leveraging to become business as usual. Every field is susceptible to this same reductionism—to putting on blinders that block out the causes and consequences of certain policies and practices. It's the assumption that what is profitable at the level of the individual account or firm will be profitable at the level of the economy as a whole. A fractal thinker would have paused before making that assumption.

Thinking fractally may sound like a readily followed prescription, but it's not easy to leave your intellectual and social comfort zone—the everyday life of the mind, which tends to everyday tasks—for reminders of where we come from and where we're going. But innovation, which will be required if you're to flourish on this crowded and unequal planet, requires such fractal thinking. It requires not forgetting connections.

It requires knowing something, too, about how our planet and our species got to be this way: it requires looking back at history. If humans have a wonderful ability to remember, we also have an unnerving ability to forget. Allow me to take as an example some of the work I've been involved in with Partners In Health and Harvard over the past year. I was in Haiti three weeks ago and know the many scars that lie upon that land: some are recent, from last year's earthquake and ongoing cholera epidemic, but many are deeply rooted in Haiti's difficult and sometimes glorious history. It would seem obvious that relief and recovery from this latest blow, which destroyed much of Haiti's urban infrastructure and killed perhaps a fifth of its civil service, should draw on deep knowledge of the place. But for many who came to help, history began the minute they stepped off the plane. It wasn't necessarily a bad thing that uninformed people of goodwill addressed the tasks at hand—direct relief of suffering—even as they sought to learn more about Haiti and its people. But many grew frustrated with the disorder and the lack of medical facilities and supplies and left as soon as it was seemly. Of course, all of us—especially the Haitians—were frustrated by the inability of such a massive humanitarian response to save more lives and house and feed the survivors.

Facing such a catastrophe, what might thinking fractally really add? It could reveal that the earthquake was not just a "natural" disaster but also a social disaster with social roots. After all, decades of shoddy construction and absent building codes had made Haiti's capital so vulnerable to a "natural" disaster in the first place. Hurricane Katrina revealed similar social fault lines on American soil: the degradation of wetlands compounded the hurricane's destructiveness; poor communities of color, because of where they lived and because of their inability to get out of town ahead of the storm, shouldered the greatest burden of damage and suffering; rebuilding proceeds unevenly. The nuclear crises in Japan are another troubling confirmation of the social footprint of "natural" disaster.

Considering the past and thinking fractally allow us to build on accumulated knowledge and experience and to discover what the theoretical biologist Stuart Kauffman has termed "the adjacent possible." In his recent book about where good ideas come from, Steven Johnson reflects on the notion:

The strange and beautiful truth about the adjacent possible is that its boundaries grow as you explore those boundaries. Each new combination ushers new combinations into the adjacent possible. Think of it as a house that magically expands with each door you open. You begin with a room with four doors, each leading to a new room that you haven't visited yet. Those four rooms are the adjacent possible. But once you open one of those doors and stroll into that room, three new doors appear, each leading to a brand new room that you couldn't have reached from your original starting point. Keep opening doors and eventually you'll have built a palace.[20]

More on palaces in a bit. But it's impossible to stand here, in an institution celebrating its 222nd such ceremony, without a certain sense of awe about the pace of innovation and the way it's shaping our world—for good and ill, but mostly, I believe, for good. One thing is sure: communication technologies and social media have opened many new avenues for discerning the connections between us and also between those who came before; they make thinking fractally a little easier.

You are stepping out into a world that is epochally different from the one I entered upon graduating from college in 1982. Even then, the adjacent possible struck me as vast, since I was lucky enough to be shown many doors and to open several of them, moving from a research laboratory to the door that opened into a class in medical anthropology, which led me to the door that opened into Haiti, which led me back to a microscope and then on to social medicine—the branch of medicine that draws most heavily on this fractal way of seeing the world, since it moves, however uneasily, between different scales: cell, tissue, organ, patient, family, society, globe.

I spent the year after my college graduation in Haiti, and it was that year that hooked me on thinking fractally because it highlighted the connections, rather than the disjunctures, of our world. I saw rural farmers unable to sell their produce because subsidized "food aid" from abroad was cheaper, local fishermen trolling depleted oceans because deforestation had silted in the reefs, a feverish democracy interrupted by foreign-backed coups and embargoes, pathogens introduced from abroad without the corresponding therapeutics. Everything seemed connected to everything. In the dormitory at Harvard Medical School, in an inscription on the ceiling, all of us could read an aphorism from the great French chemist, Louis Pasteur: "Chance favors the prepared mind." That increasingly comes to mean, as Steven Johnson reminds us, that chance favors the *connected* mind.

Communication technologies may help you tackle the ills of the social world by enabling you to harness the connections among people near and far, past and present. You have access to more information than any previous generation; the challenge before you is not just to get information, but to discern what's actually of worth since a lot of it is silly—or worse. Just in the past few months, new social media like Facebook and Twitter are credited (with some immodesty, perhaps) for helping move forward democratic change in Egypt, Tunisia, Yemen, and perhaps Libya and Syria. We shall see, and in short order.

By the way, I won't embarrass you by asking all those who have texted or tweeted during the course of this ceremony to raise their hands. But if I asked all those who rely on such forms of communication to raise their hands, only a few very old-school faculty and great-grandparents, and the rare young Luddite, would not have them up in the air. This is a Jesuit institution, not a Trappist one. A few weeks ago, a few of my medical students were waxing nostalgic about their old-school computers, and I almost stopped the conversation by noting that I once owned a typewriter. From the embarrassed silence that followed, you'd think that I'd boasted of sending missives on papyrus.

II.

Two dangers of the new social media are the erasure of history and the decline of critical analysis. It's not just that social complexity can't be captured in fewer than 140 characters. It's that facile connectivity can crowd out habits of critique. This is true in a prosaic sense: constant bombardment with communications of all sorts can eat up time that might have been spent reading and writing and reflecting. I don't mean to offer another old-school jeremiad bemoaning the decline of reading and human intelligence with every new technology; we've all heard predictions about epidemic ADD. But I also think those who herald the new social media as the latest in a triumphal parade of freedom- and knowledge-promoting innovations—from writing (my trusty papyrus) to the codex to the movable-type printing press to the Internet—may oversimplify the point. Adam Gopnik called this "the *Wired* version of Whig history."[21] Something may get lost in all the cheering: habits of critical self-reflection that are required to perceive and diagnose the many problems of the social world around us.

My second suggestion, therefore, is that you do what the Jesuits do: *cultivate an ability to look at the world critically.* Since you're graduating from Georgetown, some of you know that Catholic social teaching demands not only service to the poor (on which, more in a bit), but also discernment. Seeing and judging and acting well require careful study and reflection. We are to feed the hungry, yes, but also to ask why hunger persists (or worsens), even as global food production and distribution capacity advances. As we dig our way out of a global financial crisis that will affect your paths in the coming months and years, don't we need to reflect on Martin Luther King's argument that "True compassion is more than flinging a coin to a beggar.... [True compassion] comes to see that an edifice which produces beggars needs restructuring"?[22] How can we address these structural and socially complex problems if we don't understand them?

Allow me to give another example about Haiti. A critical and fractal view of the world might reveal a thing or two about how Haiti can "build back better" (to use Bill Clinton's optimistic phrase) in the long term. As we gather here today, reconstruction in Haiti is stalled. Long-term investments are slow to materialize. And they are desperately needed, as are shovel-ready projects that clear rubble, rebuild houses, and give paid jobs to hundreds of thousands of jobless Haitians. Of $10 billion in reconstruction aid pledged for Haiti, less than 20 percent has arrived, and very little of that has ended up in Haitian hands. A critical and long view of foreign aid reveals that donors often default on aid promises after the press release or photo op. After four hurricanes rocked Haiti in as many weeks in 2008, only 15 percent of rebuilding pledges ever made it to Haiti.

Beyond the numbers, a critical view would demand rewriting the rules of the road for foreign assistance in Haiti. The earthquake showed in high relief that the "republic of NGOs," as Haiti has been termed, has little to show after decades of NGO-driven development projects. The standard practice in foreign assistance of making aid flow to the private sector (including NGOs) while bypassing the public sector has unwittingly weakened the Haitian government. And with an anemic public sector, public health and public education were crumbling well before the quake. The cholera epidemic is the most recent instance of what happens when the public sector is neglected: no amount of private enterprise can replace a reliable public water supply. Knowledge of the history of foreign aid and its mixed results could guide a new approach in which donors and goodwill initiatives from abroad do not simply donate, but *accompany* Haitian groups in the public and private sectors to help build Haiti back better.[23]

Critical analysis—asking deep questions about root causes—reminds us that some things change while others do not. The challenge before you graduates is the challenge faced by all those blessed with opportunity: to be a positive force in a changing and connected world. When the Jesuits founded Georgetown at the close of the eighteenth century, they surely had the same idea in mind. But analytic rigor need not be the exclusive province of university faculty any more than good study habits are useful only to those enrolled as students. Reading critically is part of what will help you solve persistent problems, from hunger to reconstruction after a natural disaster to finding energy sources that do not cripple our planet further than we have already. Use your education, and also your privilege, to address the world's most pressing challenges.

III.

Third and final point: *engage in service to others.* It's not true, perhaps, that just any sort of service will do. But the list of possible ways to serve is long. One well-known alumnus of this university, who shall go unnamed but who after his graduation served two terms as president of the United States, has written a fine little book called *Giving.* He makes the same point: "All kinds of giving can make a profoundly positive difference."[24] He also makes a distinction between public service in politics and "the explosion of private citizens doing public good," and wishes he'd done more of it: "When I was in my first year of college, I gave a little time to a community project Georgetown University ran in poor neighborhoods in Washington, DC, and contributed to the occasional good cause, but I dedicated most of my free time to friends and campus activities. During my last two years of college, at Oxford, and at Yale Law School, I became obsessed with politics and gave very little time or money to anything else."[25] Does this sound familiar? Don't bother raising your hands—I know the answer.

Social progress, like innovation in general, is rarely the work of lone wolves but rather of teams. The social world is shaped by time and place and forces beyond our control. But it is also a product of the people and groups that constitute its basic fabric, and it is, therefore, also ours for the making and re-making, as long as we don't try to go it alone. One of the chief lessons from my own experience as a physician is that we can do great things when we pull together, when we are connected.

Sometimes our work in global health connects people all over the globe. After the earthquake, a Georgetown student named Natalia Moreno, who had visited us in Haiti at the close of 2009, organized fellow students here and, in a single evening, raised about $30,000 for our earthquake relief efforts. She was able to do that because she and her peers together added up to more than the sum of their parts. She even called on her brother, an artist in Bogota, to design a really cool hat, with "Here for Haiti" as the logo, which she promised to give me. All I got was a lousy mortarboard! The service ethic is not dead at Georgetown, of course; it's part of the ethos here, alive and well and waiting to be harnessed more effectively.

Some even harder tasks await, whether you are going into Teach for America or graduate school or finance. Our world, including this country, is becoming ever more unequal. I won't burden you with grim facts, but they all point to the same thing: a growing divide between the haves and the have-nots. This is not some "natural" process, but one shaped by policies and by a social environment in which it's deemed acceptable for some to have so much and others to have so little. Clinton—you guessed it—put it this way in his book on giving:

> The modern world, for all its blessings, is unequal, unstable, and unsustainable.... As long as more than 100 million children in poor countries are not enrolled in school, there will be political and social instability, with global implications. There is a growing backlash against the global economy in both rich and poor nations where the economic growth it has stimulated has not been broadly shared. About half of the world's people still live on less than $2 a day.[26]

This is not the world you want to pass on to your children, for it is a world in which fewer and fewer people have more and more chances, while the majority faces tough decisions about how to feed and educate their children and keep them safe. Such disparities can make the world an ugly and unsafe place that breeds deep resentments over the lack of readily available possibility.

To return to the adjacent possible, we want to open countless doors and create new and splendid edifices. But we don't want to build palaces in the old-school sense: ornate places to which few can repair. To strain the metaphor in closing, we need to build a lot more shared palaces, ones that draw on innovation but are available to the many. We need open-source palaces. In medicine, we've tried to do this with everything from electronic medical records to hospitals that admit every patient who walks through the front door. One ambitious project underway is a new teaching hospital—the largest we've ever helped build—in central Haiti.[27] It's our hope that this will become a grand palace of healing, and also that it will promote an appreciation for the commons—what we share, or need to share.

Perhaps I can best blend these three messages into one by quoting Dr. Martin Luther King's last sermon at Ebenezer Baptist Church, delivered shortly before he was killed. The greatest thing about King's redemptive vision is that it reminds us that each of us may, at any time, choose to place the well-being of others above our own. All of us may strive for compassion, justice, and altruism, even though we lack MLK's vision and heroism. "Everybody can be great," said Dr. King, "because anybody can serve."

Now, as our country and our world face continued financial crisis (nothing new for the poor), environmental disaster, wars, and growing inequality, is the time for you to explore the adjacent possible and to serve. It's a great time to do what many Georgetown students have already done and will continue to do: to draw on deep reserves of compassion and solidarity and, above all, to tackle together the ranking problems of our times. They are many, and they are complex, but I look out over a flowering field of Hoyas and know that the future is in good hands.

Thank you, and God bless each of you.

PART IV

Service, Solidarity, Social Justice

This last section of this book includes addresses that were difficult to write and to deliver. They touch on subjects not often discussed in medicine and public health, though they must be confronted every day in clinical practice: loss and grief, making meaning of suffering and death, consolation and solidarity. Where injury occurs often and death prematurely, these topics cannot be avoided.

My teachers and colleagues in anthropology, the discipline that has informed much of my research and writing, are the experts, if anyone is, on the ways human beings make sense of loss. But the speeches collected in Part IV don't rest on claiming expertise. They share as much with sermons as with other forms of address. Several of them were delivered outside the university and for occasions other than commencement: one was given at a theological seminary; another during a church service; and a third, inspired by a historic homily, to mark the birthday of Martin Luther King Jr.

Reflecting on suffering is not the same as responding to it, but these reflections were born of practice in difficult times. I suppose they express my wish to see analysis profitably linked to action. The questions raised here reach far beyond medicine or anthropology or public health. How might we rethink the suffering that comes from premature illness—or from poverty, its common root cause—and our responses to it? Where might one turn for inspiration and hope?

Some have invoked human rights. Another response, for me, has been theology. Although I'm sure that all of us can learn a great deal from theology in general, *liberation theology* raises the right questions for global health work. How an omnipotent God might be considered benevolent in a world of pain and evil is not my interest here. Nor do I have a better answer than most doctors for the personalized version of such reflection—Why do bad things happen to good people?—although this question is inevitably raised by all those who suffer, which is to say everyone.

Gustavo Gutiérrez, often called the father of liberation theology, has been a mentor to me for all of my adult life. As he often observes, structural violence forces us to try to make sense of suffering in our time. But we must first acknowledge that the suffering of "good people" isn't really the right place to start. Rather, it is poor, wounded, vulnerable people who can reveal the world to us. As Dietrich Bonhoeffer asked from a Nazi prison two decades before Gutiérrez helped lay the foundations of liberation theology, "Who stands fast?"

This question that Bonhoeffer and Archbishop Oscar Romero and Father Gutiérrez asked has been posed for millennia. Its significance is sapped unless we add, "Stands fast *where? Why* and with *whom?*" Bonhoeffer learned, as did his spiritual forebears two thousand years previously, the answers to these questions.

Taking the *view from below* is the only way to seek to understand our world.

Standing fast is hard work. This is especially true during war, as Bonhoeffer learned well before he was hanged, because war— "event violence," in the midst of structural violence—causes so many to suffer. War reduces the moral options we face; it makes the choices before us seem clear. Some have bemoaned the lack of clear choices today compared to those faced by the titans who lived through fascism and stood fast. This claim has been made in every conflict during the past century, sometimes with reason. Careful study shows, however, how every path laid before those whose stories we know best (and we know a fair amount about Bonhoeffer, Romero, and other martyrs) was fraught with seduction or anesthesia or deadly compromise.

Every struggle is fraught with such perils. The fight against poverty and inequality—against structural violence—is, I am persuaded, the only holy war out there. And it's a fight best fought as Bonhoeffer and Romero and Martin Luther King Jr. fought it, and as Gutiérrez fights it to this day. Their patient nonviolence, their solidarity with the poor and oppressed, speak of an even better and more pragmatic form of solidarity. We too seek to lessen violence not by taking up arms but by building schools and hospitals.

The real protagonists of the war on poverty must of course be those struggling to free themselves from it. This point was made by each of the men mentioned above; it is the thesis of Gutiérrez's *We Drink from Our Own Wells.* But the poor and oppressed— whether during the great European conflict that claimed Bonhoeffer or the civil-rights struggle that claimed MLK or the Latin American liberation struggles that claimed Romero—desperately need allies.

The poor also need people of privilege who understand their own good fortune and do not turn away from the suffering of others. The people to whom the speeches in this book are addressed are typically young and accomplished; they've been encouraged to strive for recognition; they've been socialized for success, especially their own. The quest for personal efficacy and competition with others is the topic of one of King's most well-known sermons, which affords the title for mine. To harness such strivings to the benefit of all is a task of great importance. It is not possible, or even prudent, to suppress them.

If we cannot sublimate fully our own quests for personal efficacy, what can we do to serve others and especially the most vulnerable? Understanding how the suffering of the poorest is perpetuated is not the same as fighting it. But if we believe that knowledge can inform practice—if we believe in *praxis* as pragmatic solidarity—then it is best to strive to perceive structural violence as we try to accompany the destitute sick and advance social justice.

The term "accompaniment" is more about walking together—journeying with another—than about standing fast. At the journey's beginning, we aren't always sure where the path will lead; and we're almost never sure where the end will be. Uncertainty and openness and patience and humility are inextricable from accompaniment.

When speaking about such lofty, freighted topics as social justice and solidarity, it's important to acknowledge how difficult these are to understand or measure. There's no "key performance indicator" or "process measure" to help us here. Goodness and decency and social justice and the patient accompaniment of the sick and imprisoned and despised are not so easy to put in a formula. But just because we cannot yet quantify the impact of accompaniment, or the virtues that underpin it, does not mean we can afford to postpone it for another day. In my experience, accompaniment offers the surest means of protecting against the pitfalls inherent in our quests for personal efficacy and of moving forward, however slowly, toward equity, justice, compassion, and solidarity.

Who Stands Fast?

Union Theological Seminary,
Union Medal Acceptance Speech

DECEMBER 6, 2006

Two Tuesdays ago, three Haitian coworkers, an American volunteer, and an unlucky soul looking for a ride were kidnapped at gunpoint between Port-au-Prince and Cange, the village where Ophelia and I have been working for almost 25 years. Two days later, upon payment of a ransom, they were freed.

On April 9, 1945, as Allied forces claimed victory in Germany, Dietrich Bonhoeffer was hanged in the Flossenberg concentration camp.

Although there is all the difference in the world between kidnapping and execution, between social disintegration and war, between surviving and dying, I'd like to contemplate some of Bonhoeffer's last words as we contemplate a future in which siding with and living among the poor means running risks, whether in Haiti or Rwanda or Guatemala or parts of our own country. I'd like to think about the destitute sick, of course, but also about prisoners and criminals, about what the Union Medal means today, for the two of us and for the 4,000 people who work with us.[1]

I start with Bonhoeffer because of his association with Union, and because his *Letters and Papers from Prison* remains a source of great inspiration and guidance even today. The final paragraph of an essay called "After Ten Years: A Reckoning Made at New Year 1943" has been of particular import for many of us. Under the heading "The View from Below," he writes, "There remains an experience of incomparable value. We have for once learnt to see the great events of world history from below, from the perspective of the outcast, the suspects, the maltreated, the powerless, the oppressed, the reviled—in short, from the perspective of those who suffer."[2]

This simple insight has informed Ophelia's and my work since the two of us were fortunate enough to meet in central Haiti in May 1983. At the end of that same year, I met Jim Yong Kim, whose mother is a graduate of Union. Together with Todd McCormack, who is also here tonight, Tom White, and many, many others in Haiti, we launched Partners In Health, which always seeks to take the view from below. We didn't teach this view to each other, nor did we learn it from Bonhoeffer or from the liberation theologians who have adopted it most consistently; we learned it from Haiti. Haiti and Haitians have, for over two decades, been our greatest teachers.

Since I've just returned from Haiti and since Partners In Health's largest projects are there, I'd like to ask some questions about current events, there and elsewhere, from the perspective that Haiti has instilled in us. Let me return to the kidnapping, which was not our first and, regrettably, is unlikely to be our last.

Two of our vehicles were nearing a large market town just north of Port-au-Prince. Those in the first jeep heard gunfire from an exchange between police and a group termed "bandits," or "gang members." (A policeman and an unknown number of civilians were killed then and later that night, during police reprisals.) If we'd been following our own protocol, those in the first vehicle would have signaled to those in the second that they should turn back; if we'd been following protocol, they would not have been traveling at nightfall. But all of us have trouble following protocols. And so those in the second vehicle, oblivious, were stopped at a speed bump (a fairly ridiculous addendum to a road scarred by much worse obstacles) and taken hostage by a group of young men—heavily armed though less heavily armed than the police who were shooting at them. These young men marched our coworkers into a dense thicket on the side of the road. The vehicle was abandoned, since the kidnappers knew that an American hostage was more valuable than a jeep.

Our coworkers and the hapless *woulibe*—the Haitian term for someone who hitches a free ride—spent two miserable nights under the stars. They were blindfolded and marched for hours to some sort of camp. They were threatened with guns to the head unless a ransom was paid. One of them was manhandled. All of them feared for their lives.

But since these five did have friends working hard for their release, I'd like to follow Bonhoeffer's lead and turn the story on its head, or at least tilt it slightly. Our hostages were, all told, lucky. It did not rain either night, although this is the rainy season. They were threatened with execution, but they were fed. One of the hostages was roughed up, but the others were untouched. Another, a young woman, was allowed to bathe unmolested. The hostages were robbed, but the American was given his wallet back after the ransom was paid. He decided not to look in it until later, but when he did, he found all his credit cards, if not in the sleeves in which he'd placed them. The kidnappers left him $40 and didn't touch his passport. The hostages had been blindfolded during the day but at night were able to see that a good many of those who'd captured them were teenagers. Some of the older "bandits" were hard cases; they boasted that they would use the ransom money to buy better weapons because they and their families, they said, had been victims of police brutality. At least one teenager told our friends that both his parents had been killed by security forces.

I'm not trying to make excuses for those who kidnapped my friends. I want rather to ask why such events occur at all. No-go zones cut across Port-au-Prince, just as they do in most of Brazil's major cities or parts of Johannesburg, not to mention certain U.S. cities. You can find violence almost everywhere. Some seek to understand the root causes of such criminality; others, especially in this country, have suggested that even seeking root causes of violence excuses the perpetrators. In any case, we at Partners In Health don't have the option to ignore these questions, as we must conduct our work in settings of poverty and inequality, which are, by definition, settings of violence. We've been very fortunate, so far. Although several of us have been threatened or detained, none have been killed or even seriously wounded. That's an excellent record, in Haiti. We think we've fared well in large part because we fight the violence around us not with weapons but with food, water, schools, clinics, and hospitals.

After mass two Sundays ago, this latest kidnapping was much discussed. Our American guest was a great sport about the whole thing, joking that he'd just spent two nights in "a hotel that didn't merit even three stars"—they slept on the ground—and complained that "the food was subpar." But many of my Haitian friends and patients from the village observed that the current epidemic of kidnappings—some have named Port-au-Prince the kidnapping capital of the world—was launched rather spectacularly by the kidnapping of their own president in 2004.

Are our Haitian friends and patients right? Was President Jean-Bertrand Aristide kidnapped? What we know is that the elected president of Haiti said he was taken from office against his will. His claim has been echoed by several members of the U.S. Congress and certain human rights groups. We know, too, that he was taken away on a U.S. government plane. Our soon-to-be-former Secretary of Defense dismissed this allegation as "ridiculous." Our former Secretary of State insisted that the Haitian president was flown "to a destination of his choice. . . . So this was not a kidnapping."[3] Regardless of your views on the probity of our cabinet members, it seems unlikely that the Haitian president would choose as his destination the Central African Republic, a country he had never visited, one that had its own coup d'état a few months previously, and was known for its lawlessness. (Speaking of records, the BBC had just about then dubbed Bangui, the capital of said republic, as the most dangerous city in the world.)

Haitians know a lot about kidnapping, of course. Almost all of them are descendants of people kidnapped from Africa, although pundits outside of Haiti dismiss such legacies as irrelevant. Toussaint L'Ouverture, the Haitian general who led the world's first successful slave revolt, was invited at the dawn of the nineteenth century to a parley with French forces along with the usual assurances in a negotiation between the heads of opposed armies. Instead of a parley, there was a kidnapping: L'Ouverture was chained and put on a boat bound for France, where he later died—of tuberculosis it's said—in a cold French prison.

Dietrich Bonhoeffer was arrested, rather than kidnapped, but it's likely that he saw it coming. Some of his friends here at Union certainly did: they encouraged him to remain in the States and, later, to return here until the war was over. He knew the risks and did not shirk them in returning to his family and his pastoral work. All around him, he saw German civilians, the great majority of them Jews, being kidnapped and taken away never to return. "Who stands fast?" he asked from prison.

Who stands fast? How should we know what to do in a time of war? Partners In Health is a secular organization, but all of us embrace the corporal works of mercy, laid out clearly enough in the Gospels (Matthew 25:34). These are not vague injunctions. Feed the hungry. Give drink to the thirsty. Clothe the naked. Shelter the homeless. Visit the sick. Visit the prisoners. Bury the dead.

We've had no choice but to consider these commands carefully in choosing to remain in Haiti and to expand our work in Africa, Siberia, parts of Latin America. These commands became, in fact, our guiding philosophy. One of the things that surprised us most, as Partners In Health grew, was just how contentious this philosophy was among our peers, the "experts" in international health and development. Feeding the hungry was not sustainable, we heard. Treating AIDS in Haiti was initially dismissed by some of our peers (though never by our patients) as quixotic or worse. Others said, with animus, "Surely you can't be serious about building houses for Haitian peasants with AIDS? That's not cost-effective."

Indeed, we've been lectured a lot about our work. Doctors and nurses are wasting their time doing home visits. You can't work in prisons; it's too political. You shouldn't provide Siberian prisoners with better care than is available to Russian civilians. African women with HIV are too poor to avoid breastfeeding their infants. Trying to provide clean water and formula, which would help eliminate pediatric AIDS, is not "realistic" in rural Africa. Et cetera.

Although we have tried to master the language of international health and sustainable development, and although we've learned much in doing so, I still believe we've learned more by returning to these first principles, laid out so long ago in the Gospel according to Matthew.

What have we learned? That Partners In Health is in a precarious position. We have to find the resources to feed the hungry, even when we receive funding to treat disease. We have to build schools, even when we know that the hungry children who will learn there will not be able to pay for a midday meal, which should be their right. We have to bury the dead, even if it means hiring someone to build coffins as we seek to make premature death a less prominent feature of the communities in which we work. Sometimes we have to take risks in order to exhume bodies thrown into mass graves and bury them properly, as their surviving relatives wish.

We still have to visit prisoners, whether in Sing Sing, Guantanamo Bay, Siberia, or Rwanda. If our friends' kidnappers were to end up in a squalid Haitian prison—less likely, under present circumstances, than summary execution or death in another gun battle—would we not visit them? Bring them food? How many of the hungry, sick prisoners we visited in Haiti just this past Saturday were kidnappers? We don't know. Few of them have ever been convicted of a crime; they're simply detained. And some of them need immediate medical attention in addition to the Gospel-required visit. When we bring medicines to a prisoner in eastern Rwanda, knowing that we are surrounded by more than 7,000 men who took part in their country's 1994 genocide, do we shrug and say that criminals such as these do not deserve medical care? That they are in prison *for* punishment, not *as* punishment?

In a time when habeas corpus becomes not a right but an option for the U.S. government and when "extraordinary rendition" is the latest term for kidnapping, do we shrug our shoulders and say, "Well, it's a time of war"? When the president of our nation's oldest neighbor, Haiti, is "rendered" all the way to Central Africa, do we buy into the dismissals and character assassination of the powerful, as so many in our country did? As we did regarding weapons of mass destruction in Iraq and that country's supposed links with Al Qaeda? Most of the "reasonable" people, after all, were only too happy to dismiss the latest coup d'état in Haiti, or the genocide in Rwanda, as either the result of bad third-world leadership or ethnic conflict. And "reasonable" people assured us we'd be welcomed as liberators in Iraq. Wasn't this the news as presented in our nation's papers of record?

Allow me to close with another reflection from Bonhoeffer. Under the heading, "Who Stands Fast?" he chides his peers. And his peers sound a lot like our peers, do they not? He writes:

> The "reasonable" people's failure is obvious. With the best intentions and a naïve lack of realism, they think that with a little reason they can bend back into position the framework that has got out of joint. In their lack of vision they want to do justice to all sides, and so the conflicting forces wear them down with nothing achieved. Disappointed by the world's unreasonableness, they see themselves condemned to ineffectiveness; they step aside in resignation or collapse before the stronger party.[4]

None of us can be dead sure who the "stronger party" is today. All of us would like to be considered reasonable and effective. At least tonight, no one in this room has to fear kidnapping, or worse. But doing social justice work, even in the arena of health care for the poor, brings risks; it demands that we question ourselves when we become too reasonable, when we replace what must be done with what's feasible. Partners In Health will use this award recognition to continue a ministry of simply showing up and doing the best we can do. You are honoring us, we believe, because we have questioned and resisted the proffered wisdom about what might be accomplished among and for the poorest of the poor.

We'll take risks if we have to. We'll be unreasonable, shrill even, if that is what is required to carry out the corporal works of mercy among the poorest. Neither of us would ever dare promise that we'd have Bonhoeffer's courage if faced with prison or worse. But the recognition we've received tonight from people we've long admired inspires us to continue in these works and to hope for the courage to avoid becoming worn down, condemned to ineffectiveness. And even as we expand our projects, sometimes we hope only to hold fast.

Thank you for this great honor.

Courage and Compassion in the Time of Guantánamo

Emory University, Commencement

MAY 14, 2007

Forgive me, dear graduates and families and friends, if I'm a bit intimidated about being your commencement speaker. I consider it a great honor, of course, but you'll have to admit there's been a fair amount of flak about this part of the festivities. I'm accustomed to being second choice and don't mind losing out to major contributors to higher education, such as Will Ferrell or the Rock.

In any case, friends here have sent me copies of the editorials and letters in your campus newspaper, the *Wheel*. So I know that Emory is at least polite about such matters as who should give your commencement address. When the president of George Washington University was announced as the commencement speaker at that institution, I read, again in your newspaper, that he

> was labeled a "con artist" and a "spawn of Satan" on Facebook groups created to protest his decision. At Emory, students maintained their respect for Wagner while protesting his decision.
>
> The Emory administration was also able to respond to student concerns with a greater deal of success. Commencement at George Washington will continue without a keynote speaker. . . .

> Emory, on the other hand, was able to recruit an outside speaker, Paul Farmer, who, while not widely recognized by students, at least fits the ideals of the University he will be addressing.

So here I am, not recognized by anyone here and not as appealing as a celebrity or a political figure. But even the *Wheel* offers hope that I might have something useful to impart and has been kind enough not to publish any Facebook commentaries suggesting that it is I who am the spawn of Satan. Good news for me.

And some good news for you: my remarks will be brief, contain a true story with a plotline, and attempt to reflect some of the ideals that Emory, as much as any research university, is attempting to cultivate. I will try to avoid focusing only on the dreary topics in which I have, alas, some expertise. Oh, don't worry: I wouldn't know how to give a speech without referring to runaway epidemics and pestilence in general; to war, racism, and other sorts of violence. I wouldn't know how not to speak about people I've met by being a doctor. But, since today is the day of your commencement, I will try to discuss these horrors in a cheerful way.

So I'm going to tell a story about one family's struggle.

I.

It's a story about courage and commitment, friendship and generosity. It's a story about immigration to this country, and it links, in no more than a dozen years, four very different countries. It's a story that leads from Haiti to the United States via Guantánamo, where we have a military base, and then on to Iraq. Four countries, twelve years. I said I wouldn't be talking about the war much, and I won't. I said I wouldn't talk too much about disease and violence, and I won't. I will focus on a courageous and generous young man, whom I'll call "Joe" since he's still in Iraq. He's about the same age as many of you graduating today. I've told his mother's story before, but his, never before today.

I met Joe because of a 1991 military coup d'état in Haiti, where I'd been working since graduating from college. Joe's parents were poor but able to read and write and interested in service to others. They were deeply involved in a mass literacy movement that had taken root in Haiti around the time of that country's first democratic elections, which occurred in December 1990. Seven months after a landslide victory brought a liberation theologian to the presidency and more resources to bear on Haiti's stubborn poverty, a violent military coup brought an end to democratic rule in Haiti. The ensuing repression was fearsome. Refugees streamed out of the cities and into the hills, over the border into the Dominican Republic (where they were unwelcome), and onto the high seas.

Of course no one desired to leave home, least of all a young couple with two small boys. But on April 27, 1992, Joe's mother, Yolande Jean, was arrested and taken to a police station. Yolande, visibly pregnant with her third child, was beaten. On her second day in prison, she miscarried. She did not receive medical attention and decided that, if she survived detention, she would flee the country. She was released from prison the following day. Shortly thereafter, she entrusted her sons to a kinswoman and headed for northern Haiti. Her husband remained in hiding, and she did not see him again.

The next part of the story brings in two more of the four countries: the United States and Cuba. Why Cuba? Because that's where a U.S. Coast Guard cutter took Yolande. This is how she described it:

> I took the boat on May twelfth, and on the fourteenth they came to get us. They did not say where they were taking us. We were still in Haitian waters at the time.... We hadn't even reached the Windward Passage when American soldiers came for us. But we thought they might be coming to help us ... there were sick children on board. On the fourteenth, we reached the base at Guantánamo.[5]

Haiti was full to overflowing with people like Yolande Jean. Soon Guantánamo was full to overflowing as well. On May 24, 1992, President Bush issued Executive Order 12,807 from his summer home in Kennebunkport. Referring to the Haitian boats, he ordered the Coast Guard "to return the vessel and its passengers to the country from which it came ... provided, however, that the Attorney General, in his unreviewable discretion, may decide that a person who is a refugee will not be returned without his consent." As an attorney for the Lawyers Committee for Human Rights wryly observed, "Grace did not abound; all Haitians have been returned under the new order."[6]

Not all were returned: Yolande was among that small number who, deemed political refugees, were also found to be positive for HIV. I won't go through her whole story, which is too painful for a day of celebration like this one, but suffice it to say she was detained and mistreated. The plight of Haitian refugees became enough of a cause célèbre during the 1992 elections to spur the candidates Clinton and Gore, in their official platform, to call for an end to forced repatriation of Haitian boat people and to the detention of HIV-positive refugees in Guantánamo. I'm for that, I thought, taking heart, for I was horrified by the reports coming out of our military base there. But the camps were not closed down until federal judge Sterling Johnson heard the case brought against the U.S. government by the Haitians and their advocates. The more depositions he heard, the more convinced he became that the detention of the HIV-positive Haitians represented "cruel and unusual punishment" in violation of the Eighth Amendment of the U.S. Constitution. In his 1993 ruling on the case, Judge Johnson described Haitians detained in Camp Bulkeley as follows:

> They live in camps surrounded by razor barbed wire. They tie plastic garbage bags to the sides of the building to keep the rain out. They sleep on cots and hang sheets to create some semblance of privacy. They are guarded by the military and are not permitted to leave the camp, except under military escort. The Haitian detainees have been subjected to pre-dawn military sweeps as they sleep by as many as 400 soldiers dressed in full riot gear. They are confined like prisoners and are subject to detention in the brig without hearing for camp rule infractions.[7]

Yolande was duly released, along with the others, to cities in the United States. I visited her and other Haitian refugees in New York and Boston after this particular ordeal was over. When I first met Joe, he was about twelve; his brother, ten. I mostly talked to their mom and seem to recall that they found it more absorbing to talk to my brother, who was then a professional wrestler with World Championship Wrestling and thus himself a resident of this city and a frequent visitor to Emory. (Some of you will recall that whenever I'd come here to give a talk, he'd get all the attention from my nerdy friends on the faculty. Not that I'm jealous.)

A decade went by, and I confess I didn't think much about Joe. But just before Christmas 2005 I received, via a close friend of his, a check for $250. Joe said he wished to support the work of our group, Partners In Health, in Haiti and to help us one day in serving the destitute sick there.

I was grateful for the contribution, for we certainly needed the help in Haiti. What struck me most, though, was that Joe was in Fallujah. He'd joined the Marines and been sent to Iraq.

I wrote back to him, and we stayed in touch through email and, once in a while, by phone. (Those Halliburton call centers do work, I guess, although heaven knows how high the bills are.) For a year, we corresponded almost every day, but we didn't talk much about the war or his daily reality. He took great pains to let me know that, by the time I began inquiring anxiously about his safety, he no longer went out on missions "beyond the wire," but was responsible for supplying another group of Marines out on patrol. More often than not, he'd tell me that I was the one who needed to be careful, since he knew what was happening in Haiti. But I could tell that being in Iraq was a great struggle for him—an outward and an inward struggle. I knew that he was distressed by what he was hearing about Guantánamo, and had to assume he was thinking about his own mother's experience there.

Once, when I sent him a care package, I weighed carefully what sort of books to include. Something light, I thought. "No," he said by email, "send me things about Haiti. Like I told you, I want to go back to Haiti one day and work with you." And so I sent him one of my own books about Haiti, concerned that he might find my detailed description of his mother's experience harrowing.[8] He didn't say one way or another, but after he read it, he asked me to send a copy to a friend of his. "He's Native American," wrote Joe. "He'll like it." And he reiterated his offer to come and volunteer in our clinics in Haiti.

Over a year of brief but almost daily emails, our connection deepened. When, last month, Joe returned to see his mother, brother, and girlfriend, we made plans to meet. Any city, any time, I said: I'll take you out for a nice meal and we'll catch up.

I was in Haiti when Joe wrote me one Monday. It was nighttime in Fallujah, and he was leaving just then for the States; he'd call me as soon as he landed.

My phone rang on Saturday, and shortly thereafter I got to enjoy a long reunion with Joe, meet his girlfriend, and see his brother briefly. Joe allowed, during the course of a long meal that included what I reckoned to be the first red wine he'd had in a while, that the main reasons he was planning to stay in Iraq were to look after his mother, who he knew might fall ill at any time; to send his brother to a proper college; and to be able to buy a home and have a family. "I want to look forward, not back," said the irrepressibly optimistic Joe. Some things we didn't discuss, including the fact that Joe is not yet a U.S. citizen. But we did discuss his brother's plans. Whenever he had trouble making ends meet, Joe's brother thought about joining the military too. "Do that only as a last resort," advised Joe. "I'll find the money for you to finish college." There was so much left to talk about that we talked on the phone just about every day during his leave. He is now back in Fallujah, and I spoke with him yesterday, after arriving here for commencement.

II.

So what, exactly, is this story about? What, as we used to say in medical school, is the take-home message?

Let me offer three. First, it's a story about *connections*. As you head off to lives full of promise, remember that the connections you've made here at Emory need to be sustained and nourished. I let Joe fall out of my life for a decade, and his mother and brother too. Thankfully, Joe's generosity brought us all back together. I won't lose track of them again; friendship is too precious a gift.

There are of course other, less sentimental connections visible in this story. I've written reams about the intimate links between my country and Haiti, this hemisphere's two oldest republics. It's not the stuff of congratulatory addresses, either. And the connection between our country and Iraq will cause us grief, I fear, for generations. Fallujah is a case in point and already a proverb. Just two weeks ago, one U.S. colonel in Anbar province explained his approach to counterinsurgency: "Fix Ramadi, but don't destroy it. Don't do a Fallujah."[9]

But what about our peculiar military base in, of all places, Cuba? Just last month, a friend of mine gave a talk about Gitmo at Harvard. Here's his description of the place:

> A bay, a harbor, a hideout, a home, a military base, a sanctuary, a prison; an outpost on the threshold of nations where neither Cuban, nor U.S., nor international law applies.... Guantánamo Bay has been there all along—when the Taino Indians met Columbus, when Caribbean pirates preyed on the shipping of newly consolidated states, when Spain clashed with Britain, when the U.S. defeated Spain, when Kennedy confronted Castro, when George W. Bush set out to vanquish terror. To know Guantánamo is to know ourselves—as citizens, as a country, as individuals in a world of states.[10]

Guantánamo is a place outside the reach of constitutional protections, so you might think of it as a place of disconnection. But the very disconnection connects you and me to that place and what is done there. It's a denial of responsibility, and like all such denials, it won't hold up forever. I hope you will all take on the responsibility of remembering how closely we are connected to the things that should disquiet us.

I know one should avoid Latin turns of phrase in commencement speeches, but I'm going to cheat and quote Cicero: "Not to know what happened before one was born is always to be a child."[11] As you go out into the world, remember this injunction, which Susan Sontag echoed sharply two millennia later:

> Someone who is perennially surprised that depravity exists, who continues to feel disillusioned (even incredulous) when confronted with evidence of what humans are capable of inflicting in the way of gruesome, hands-on cruelties upon other humans has not reached moral or psychological adulthood. No one after a certain age has the right to this kind of innocence, of superficiality, to this degree of ignorance, or amnesia.[12]

Second point: Joe's story, like his mother's, is for me a parable that begs the question: what kind of country do we want to live in? Look around you. Look at the way Emory looks today compared to the way it looked only 50 years ago. You know, probably, that Emory was founded in the first half of the nineteenth century by people who owned slaves. But did you know that Emory was forbidden by state law from educating African Americans at the same time it enrolled white students? Did you know that it was only in 1962, when about half of those present today were already alive, that Emory brought suit against the state of Georgia and won the right to enroll students without regard to race?

How do you want Emory to look in the future? I have a friend who's a journalist at CNN and lives right here in this city, and I asked him what points he thought I should underline today. Every day he has to read about Iraq, shooting sprees on college campuses, and crude comments from talk show hosts with followings in the millions. "It's about respecting people," he said, "and reaching out to others." He paused a second and added, "If everyone around you looks exactly like you, there's something wrong."

Although our elite universities are less homogeneous than they were a couple decades ago, they remain islands of privilege with far too few people like Joe. And although his younger brother has aspirations to attend a decent college, it's unlikely he could transfer here from the community college he now attends, especially given that he's working an almost full-time job on top of his studies. (Remember, sending money home is one of the main reasons Joe is staying in Iraq.) But still: look around you and wonder what this place would look like if we were not a country of immigrants. We ought to be celebrating this heritage with gratitude. But one can read in this month's *Harper's* Index that no fewer than 305 new U.S. anti-immigration groups have formed since January 2005.[13]

What kind of place do we want our country to be? I ask this knowing that not everyone here is a U.S. citizen. Then again, neither is Joe, even though he's serving in Iraq. If you're here today you are somehow part of this country, this great experiment in modern democracy. Granted, our nation's reputation is not impeccable: consider slavery, as noted, and the genocide of Native Americans. But until quite recently the United States has often served as a beacon of hope in many parts of the world. How do we wish to be seen by others? Or, to refer again to the *Wheel*, what are the ideals we hold dear? Do we want America to be a place that sanctions and outsources torture? Do we want to have camps like those on Guantánamo, which have been used in the struggle against Haitian refugees and also in an endless "war on terror"? Do we want America to be a place known as violent at home and violent abroad?

Third, *remember people like my uncomplaining, brave, and generous friend Joe.* I know some of the reasons he's in Fallujah rather than in Haiti or in New York, and I think you do too. The forces that tore his family asunder and sent his mother to an "HIV-positive concentration camp" are not unrelated to those that would ten years later lead him to Iraq. If you're the praying sort, please pray for Joe and for all those souls who, regardless of nationality, now find themselves within the borders of Iraq.

But the reason I mention Joe today is his generosity. In the midst of all that he's been through, he's still able to think about service to others, including people in the poverty-stricken country he has not seen since he was a child. Even in Iraq, Joe is still able to remember those less fortunate than himself. These are worthy ideals, and not unrelated, I suspect, to the kinds of service for which Emory stands. There is, in your students and faculty, enormous promise for the world in which we live.

The *Wheel's* recent editorial about today's festivities concludes, "We hope the Commencement ceremonies give our graduates a send-off to remember." I know *I* won't forget your allowing me to share this day with you and am grateful for the chance to reflect about connections visible and invisible, about the need to remember the less fortunate, even from a place like Iraq, and about the importance of service in transforming this world into a better place for all of us. I don't doubt that some of you in the audience today have reached this milestone after a journey not unlike Joe's, a passage across national borders, over class lines, through hardship and adjustment. It wouldn't surprise me to learn that Emory has inspired and shaped all of you—those who came here with all the advantages no less than those who came here with few. That is part of the utopia that gives our country its meaning, that gives the university based on research and teaching its value.

As you go forth from these extraordinary years of freedom and discovery, I ask you to keep alive in your minds the curiosity that brought you here and to revive it from time to time by forging new connections to others who would have done well with the same opportunities, had they been so fortunate.

Congratulations on the outcome of your hard work, the support of your families and friends, and on your desire to improve. Thank you for the honor of sharing this day with you.

Spirituality and Justice

All Saints Parish (Brookline, MA), Spirituality and Justice Award Acceptance Speech

APRIL 27, 2008

I am very grateful for this award and for the chance to speak to you. It's somewhat conventional to open remarks, whenever awards are concerned, with disclaimers. Here is mine: I'm pretty sure I don't deserve an award for spirituality and justice. As one person in a huge team seeking to promote basic rights for those living in poverty, I shouldn't be singled out in such a manner. No one can promote justice on his own. The Partners In Health team, thousands strong, promotes justice by making pragmatic interventions designed to bring health care, education, and clean water to the poorest.

There are other reasons that lead me to worry about the quality of my own spirituality: as an American in the time of war and water-boarding and Guantánamo, I find that my faith, both in humanity and in God, is shaken every day. As an anthropologist, I was trained to look at religions, rituals, and spiritualities of all sorts in sociological terms as universally encountered "belief systems" or cosmologies. As a reader, my favorite book on spirituality is a novel about a cloistered Catholic nun whose spiritual life is completely arid until she starts having blinding migraines and becomes, in a short space of time, a celebrated poet of spirituality. She is later found to have a brain tumor and then must ask questions about the origins of her newfound faith. (To my delight, I learned that this beautiful novella, *Lying Awake*, was written by a good Jewish boy.) As someone who has long worked in Haiti, I've lost two friends in recent years. One of them, human-rights activist Lovinsky Pierre-Antoine, is still officially "missing." Yet I have little faith that he is still alive. All these experiences make it hard to say blandly and without qualifications that the world is run by a triple complex of justice, power, and love.

Often enough, I find it hard to disagree with Albert Einstein, who famously referred to himself as "a deeply religious nonbeliever." But he also wrote this:

> I have never imputed to Nature a purpose or a goal, or anything that could be understood as anthropomorphic. What I see in Nature is a magnificent structure that we can comprehend only very imperfectly, and that must fill a thinking person with a feeling of humility. This is a genuinely religious feeling that has nothing to do with mysticism.[14]

Richard Dawkins has been blisteringly critical of people who "cherry-pick" quotations from Einstein to support arguments regarding the existence of God.[15] To draw on popular parlance, I won't go there.

Instead, I would like to say that I, like Einstein, see in "Nature" a magnificent structure. This spirituality, if that's what it is, I can draw on always: when seeing the sick human body recover quickly with modern medicine, or, more conventionally, when contemplating the awe-inspiring view from the volcanic mountains of northern Rwanda, or a towering redwood in California, or the astounding wildlife in Maasailand, or the beauty of koi in a garden which, though made by human hands, is surely a genuflection to nature.

The example of a garden leads me to speak of another spirituality, encountered in some of the most unlovely places in the world. Now I will paraphrase Einstein and, I'd guess, part ways with him: what I sometimes see in *humanity* is a magnificent structure we can comprehend only imperfectly, and although it has nothing to do with mysticism, observing this structure fills me with a sense of humility and wonder and renewed faith.

I'll give an example from an unlovely place: inside Rwanda's largest prison. Not the first place you might go for a big dose of spirituality or justice. But there you have it: in prisons you can learn not only about crime and cruel punishment, but also about atonement, forgiveness, and—if you're lucky—about the humane treatment of people who have done terrible things.

Just three weeks ago, I was within the high, orange-bricked walls of Nsinda prison to see patients. The first time I went into this blighted place, in 2005, there were 13,000 men and a few hundred women crammed into a very small space. Although there were no juveniles in prison, infants were born there every few days. Of the adults, over 70 percent had been arrested on genocide-related charges. The place was so crowded with prisoners stacked in makeshift bunks under huge, mildewed, and dilapidated tents that it looked like a Hieronymus Bosch painting of hell. The smells were unpleasant. I knew, as any doctor would, that epidemics of tuberculosis, cholera, hepatitis, and other problems were sure to follow such overcrowding in the absence of modern sanitation.

Today, there are less than half as many in the prison, although it remains Rwanda's largest. To be precise, there were 6,334 prisoners as of April 3, 2008. How, after a genocide, do you halve the population of a prison without promoting impunity? As noted, the majority of the detainees were there on genocide-related charges. There had to be a lot of guilty parties in this crime. Best estimates are that, in the 100 days following April 6, 1994, a million Rwandans were killed upon government orders. It is thought that some 14–17 percent of the adult male Hutu population followed orders to kill all those identified as Tutsis and also Hutus considered "soft," that is, sympathetic to the plight of those targeted for death.

After a genocide, the task of a successor government is to restore not only order but also a sense of justice. If we do the math, it's easy to see that even with 200,000 in prison, as was true before the amnesties, many of the guilty must have been walking free. This was Rwanda's dilemma: to warehouse the guilty is expensive and, from the point of view of an infectious-disease physician, dangerous. To allow them to walk free, to leave them in impunity, is an offense to justice, to the memories of the victims and the feelings of their surviving kin.

How to resolve this dilemma? Many people in my circles praise what is loosely termed the "truth and reconciliation process." But the process that occurred in South Africa, for example, required courtrooms with electricity, lawyers with access to books and computers, and a legal system that, although deeply tainted by apartheid, could claim at least a few independent judges. No such resources existed in Rwanda after the genocide and very few exist today. Nsinda prison, even with 13,000 detainees, had not a single doctor on staff and only one nurse. Food procurement alone was a challenge that would, I'm sure, overwhelm any of us.

One of the ways that the Rwandan government has confronted this challenge—what to do with the guilty—has been to revive the traditional institution of *gacaca* courts. The name means, roughly, "grassy justice" because aggrieved parties are supposed to meet with village elders and air their problems publicly, sitting in a circle on the ground. In post-genocide Rwanda, almost anyone in good standing who wished to go through a training course could become a *gacaca* judge. (I know a cook, an auxiliary nurse, and a peasant farmer who are judges.) Some say up to 250,000 people have gone through this training. These al fresco courts do not handle the gravest of genocide-related crimes but do handle the great majority of them. In the practice of these courts, public atonement for misdeeds is the surest way to avoid or shorten prison sentences and end up doing community service instead. Such avowals offer prisoners their best chance of getting out of prison, too. Public involvement is close to mandatory, and a few of Rwanda's 30 districts have already completed the *gacaca* process. I know this because in one of the places we work, we were given the tribunal building and are transforming it into a hospital. Tuesday is *gacaca* day in Rwinkwavu, the place I've spent most of my time, and many activities slow to a crawl when the court is meeting.

How do the accused reach, physically, the places in which they killed? The places in which their victims and the relatives of their victims live? How do the accused avoid becoming the victims of assaults and revenge killings on the way to put in their appearance? It's the job of the prison system to escort prisoners between the prisons and the *gacaca* courts. Sometimes, when the prisoners must face their victims or their kin in an area far from where they are detained, they stay in guarded facilities on the way back to these towns and villages. One of my coworkers, Naomi Rosenberg, was visiting Rwanda for the first time this past month and was in the prison when I last saw patients there. She asked the soft-spoken warden if any of the prisoners had been harmed during this transfer process. "Not a single one since I've been here," replied the director of Rwanda's largest prison, who'd been working in the system for years. Others from outside the system admit that the entire process has been largely non-violent, in spite of expert predictions, many of them from "the international human rights community," that the *gacaca* process was doomed to fail.

That same day, I saw a couple of patients, both suffering from AIDS and tuberculosis and complications of therapy. I've worked for well over a decade in prisons in Siberia, Haiti, and Rwanda, and it has never been my practice to ask prisoners about their crimes or alleged misdeeds even though the duration of our therapies—many months for TB and a lifetime for AIDS— does require me to ask about the duration of their sentences. On that day, I did so in both instances. One of the patient-prisoners was a man I'd met before his arrest. I'd seen him a couple of times in the hospital and in the clinic in Rwinkwavu. He'd been sentenced to fifteen years, but his case, he told me, was on appeal. I asked how long it would be before his appeal would be heard. "Maybe a couple of months," he replied. I thought of some of the prisoners I'd seen in the States, where appeals take many years, or in Haiti, where the vast majority of prisoners have never even been tried and sentenced: they're simply detainees. (A moment ago, I mentioned my missing friend Lovinsky. He was one of those seeking to improve the execrable conditions of Haitian prisons.)

The other man I saw that day had been in prison since the genocide and so had served, he said, almost fourteen of the nineteen years to which he had been sentenced. I didn't have to ask anything more. I only asked about his sentence because he had AIDS and was now slated to receive what's called a "retreatment" regimen for TB, which was longer and also required us to alter his AIDS regimen.

But I had, of course, my own private and unspoken questions.

Later that day, we shared a meal with the prison director and two of the nurses. (Although we are still the only doctors who go into the prison, there are now four nurses.) The director knew the older man pretty well, which is surprising given the sheer numbers inside the prison. "He's one of the few who refuses to admit that he did anything wrong," the warden said. "That's why he's likely to serve out his sentence."

I thought just then about Lovinsky, who has tried so hard to support, in Haiti, a legal system that rejects impunity and favors human rights. Lovinsky believed, *believes*, in this vision so much that he was almost certainly willing to give his life for it—and I say this in praying that he did not.

I said already that Lovinsky's fate, whatever it may be, has led me to question my own faith. But a few days later, as I continued to contemplate my Haitian friend's fate from rural Rwanda, I found myself in a jeep between a town called Butaro, where we are building a hospital in a large region that has none, and Rwinkwavu, where we rebuilt a hospital abandoned after the genocide. At the wheel was a young man named Thierry, and I was the only passenger. He'd been born in exile in neighboring Burundi and returned after the genocide. Conversations about such matters cannot be expected to flow except in private, and even then not always. But sometimes, in long drives like this one, there comes a torrent of feeling and a story, almost always about 1994. I felt honored that Thierry shared his with me. On that ride, I learned that all four of his grandparents were killed during the genocide, as were most of his uncles and aunts and cousins and as was, most painfully to Thierry, his older brother, away at school in Rwanda in 1994. Almost his entire family was wiped out in less than a month.

I didn't say much while Thierry spoke, asking only a few questions. Among the astounding things this young man told me was the following: that during the *gacaca* process in Butare, where his brother died, he decided to go and speak to the man who had killed him.

"You decided to go to the prison?" I asked. "Why?"

"I found that when I tried to pray, I had not forgiven the man who killed my brother. I hadn't forgiven any of them. And I started to ask myself how I could speak to God through prayer if I was unable to forgive. I prayed about it a lot and decided to go to the prison to speak to him." Thierry wanted to see if he could forgive this man face to face. He had been no more than nineteen at the time.

Of course I asked Thierry what the man said. "He said he was sorry. Very sorry. And that the government had made him do it."

Thierry said he forgave the man right then and there.

It has been my great good fortune to meet, again and again over the past 25 years, so many people who restore my tattered faith. In a world in which a war in Iraq can be launched on the basis of lies missed by the watchdog agencies and by the journalists who are supposed to expose the lies of politicians, I have met people like Thierry. In a world in which very powerful nations, including mine, can conspire to overturn popular democracy in Haiti, I have met people like Lovinsky Pierre-Antoine.

In a world in which complex medical services are deemed "not cost-effective" for the poor, I have met nurses and surgeons from Brigham and Women's Hospital who perform, as they did last month, free open-heart surgery in Rwanda. In a world in which the public good is undermined by the privatization of what should be considered basic services to which all humans should have rights, I get to work with people who believe that a public hospital in rural Africa should have beautiful grounds— even koi ponds—and clean spaces as well as supplies and trained personnel and free care for all who walk through its doors. I get to work with genocide survivors willing to help rebuild clinics inside a prison full of those responsible for the mass killings that resulted in the deaths of their families.

There: I am back to a spirituality that draws on the world around us, with all its fragile and threatened beauty, and not on the worst that we humans can do to each but rather the best. Instead of vengeance, cruelty, and indifference, the spirituality of justice leads us down a different path. What can we do to restore, to rebuild, a broken world? What can we do to promote peace and beauty in a world in which the poor especially are exposed to violence and endless affront?

These are rhetorical questions, of course, but they are as spiritual as they are pragmatic.

I will close by noting that they are fundamentally questions of justice. I confess that I have long been more comfortable with questions of justice than with the topic of spirituality. That is because I have seen notions of faith and spirituality perverted in our affluent and often imperial country, a country in which unjust wars are waged and even called "Crusades." I have felt alienated from faith as it is portrayed in our country.

So I was stumped as to how to close this sermon when I wrote it en route from Rwanda to the United States. But just last week, upon returning, I received a book sent to me by Jim Wallis, an evangelical preacher who terms himself a progressive. I read his book, *The Great Awakening*, over the past few days, and it helped me reconcile my doubts about our right to invoke faith and spirituality in a world of great injustice. "The Religious Right is over," writes Wallis with what I hope is warranted confidence, "but the revival may be just beginning—a revival of justice."[16] His theology eased my angst: "Two of the great hungers in our world today are the hunger for spirituality and the hunger for social justice. The connection between the two is the one the world is waiting for, especially the new generation. And the first hunger will empower the second."[17]

Unless we link our spirituality to justice and to the good works we know to be necessary in a world in which a billion people go without adequate food, clean water, health care, and a modicum of justice, we will have, as was noted two thousand years ago, nothing but dead faith.

I share your optimism about the sea change now before us and about the possibility of a spirituality of justice and equality and am honored to be here today.

Thank you.

Making Hope and
History Rhyme

Princeton University, Commencement

JUNE 1, 2008

It's an unconventional opening gambit, outside of a courtroom, to ask for your sympathy. But, really: was it absolutely necessary to have me compete with Steven Colbert? Please don't tell me that all the students wanted Colbert and that I've been imposed on you by the faculty and administration. Last year, Seamus Heaney had to follow Bill Clinton, but Heaney is a Nobel Prize–winning poet, and both have the gift of gab. Since this is Princeton, and not the small community-based college where I teach, I'm not surprised that an academic rather than an entertainer was chosen as commencement speaker. But it makes me nervous, humbled, to be one of the last people you'll hear before you walk through the Fitz-Randolph Gate. In other words, I'm taking this privilege seriously—though I've no doubt that Harvard's speaker, who invented quidditch and Hogwarts and is said to have gone from welfare mom to become the richest woman in England, will also have the jitters.

So there you have it: in order to please you all, I'll have to be as poetic as Heaney, as funny as Colbert, as engaging as Clinton, as creative as J.K. Rowling (who, looking around these parts, may well have based Hogwarts on Princeton), and as concise as a haiku poet.

There are other reasons for you to be nice to me: as the proud holder of an honorary degree from Princeton, I've technically been a member of this remarkable family since 2006, which is why I'm wondering why no one put an orange tie in my room. Also, I will make my comments brief in the hopes that my message is not effaced completely by last night's and tonight's revelry: the haggard look today is because Palmer House was shaken for hours by what I assume were fireworks rather than surface-to-air missiles.[18]

Also to honor Princeton, I will make a tribute to the 2006 speaker by quoting one of Heaney's famous and stirring poems:

> History says, Don't hope
> on this side of the grave.
> But then, once in a lifetime
> the longed for tidal wave
> of justice can rise up,
> and hope and history rhyme.[19]

That, dear graduates, is what you need to do in order to save our fragile, beautiful, threatened world. You need to make hope and history rhyme. And, as part of a broader movement now stirring, you can. I know it.

Since I'm a doctor and an anthropologist, I might be expected to offer a prescription for this utopian vision. But I can't. What I can do today is to offer a vision of what this country and this world might look like if we work together to make it a better, kinder place, and outline the sort of efforts that will be necessary to make sure that you, dear Class of 2008, don't end up ruling a violent world of haves and have-nots. So that you don't have to wall yourselves off from the hungry and the sick, who are, along with students, my constituency. So that you don't have to hear terms like "pre-emptive war" or "collateral damage" or "terrorism" when you turn on a television. That's where we are heading, and we need to change course.

Improbably, I got this idea—this vision thing—from John McCain, surely the only idea I've ever copped from him. I was recently holed up in a hotel room, staring at a blank computer screen with only the word "Princeton" on it, and watching CNN. This is not, in principle, a smart approach to writing a speech, but inspiration comes in strange forms. The venerable presidential candidate was giving a speech, in Ohio I think, and offered a vision of what our country might look like after his first term in office. (As an aside, there are medical terms for these "visions," and there are medicines to treat them, but I know it's against the rules to be partisan in a commencement address.)

So imagine you are coming back to Princeton for your twentieth-year reunion. What would the world look like if hope and history have started to rhyme?

Don't worry: Princeton will still be named the nation's best university every year and so the *U.S. News and World Report* rankings, in 2028, will simply be assessing "colleges and universities other than Princeton." President Tilghman will be begging to go back to her lab, having raised $15 trillion dollars so that the ratio of endowment to the student body will be, oh, $100 million per student. But no one will let her get back to her test tubes. Tuition at Princeton will have gone the way of early admissions. The faculty-student ratio will still look the same at first glance but will in fact be reversed: students will each have their own little personal faculty of a dozen senior professors, available at all times, just to them. Most undergraduates will have published extensively by the time they're juniors; 45 percent will hold patents for discoveries made here and then make these discoveries available to all those who need them. Even teaching fellows will need at least two PhDs in order to address undergraduates in a classroom. Nixon's nose will still be Nixon's nose and will remain, according to my crystal ball, hole number sixteen in Princeton's storied ultimate Frisbee competition. The eating clubs will still be here, of course, but more open, and will have tasting menus prepared by French chefs called *biqueurs*. (Do I do my research, or what?)[20]

But what about the world beyond this blessed oasis? If hope and history start to rhyme, if that longed-for tidal wave of justice has washed over us, the world will be a different and better place. What might it look like?

The word "justice" is used in varied and often contradictory ways. Some of us see two broad and potentially complementary justice movements that are growing every day: the environmental movement and the social justice movement. Although they count tens of millions of adherents, they too often pay no attention to each other. Should they become truly complementary, should they take root and grow in our country and in others, then the world will be, I'm convinced, changed for the better. It could be transformed not in a haphazard way—for change is coming, dear seniors—but in the just ways desired by many of those graduating today.

What about environmental justice? I can only imagine what new technological advances will have come to pass by 2028. Our economy will be green in this utopian vision, our carbon footprint tiny compared to the bad old days when oil hit $250 a barrel in 2010, provoking, at long last, a serious commitment to alternative, clean fuels. So too for India and China, which by 2020 will have become the world's largest economies. The planet's population will have grown, of course, but at nothing like the rates we're seeing now: the human herd will no longer be culled by epidemic disease or by war. For the first time in a century, the Amazon rain forest will be growing, not shrinking. Ivory-billed woodpeckers will be commonly sighted across the southeastern United States, and several other species feared extinct will re-emerge. Peace will have settled in the Congo, sparing hundreds of thousands of lives, and thousands of mountain gorillas will munch bamboo contentedly on that side of the border, as they do today in peaceful Rwanda. Haiti will have pioneered green technologies, and half of the country will at last be reforested as poor people there will no longer be forced to cut down trees to cook meals for their families. Food security will blossom in Haiti as erosion is slowed and as U.S. and European agricultural subsidies are abandoned as unfair and counterproductive. The farm bill will be stored in a museum. There will still be snow and ice on the top of Mount Kilimanjaro, just as Greenland will still be white with glaciers, and Iceland will remain green. Neither Florida nor Bangladesh will be under water.

And as for justice? Our own nation will have acknowledged that justice is not and never was blind and taken steps toward shrinking our prison population, which is in 2008 the largest, per capita, in the world. In twenty years, we'll have found alternatives to incarceration and fought racism within the justice system. All those companies now making a killing on the privatization of prisons will have gone out of business. Many of the erstwhile inhabitants of our prisons will have good green-collar jobs as our country transforms its economy.

The death penalty will have been abolished, not just here but in China and elsewhere, and our country will have joined the International Criminal Court just as we signed on to the Kyoto Accords. Harold and Kumar, having gone to White Castle via Princeton, will no longer be able to go to Guantánamo except as tourists, since the U.S. base there will have been shuttered and transformed into a botanical garden. There will be no travel restrictions to that island.

Across the globe, torture will be well and truly outlawed. "Water-boarding" will be a term used to refer to a beachside amusement indulged in by happy kids who are not obese and diabetic, as so many were by 2010 and through no fault of their own. There will still be a show called *24*, but it will be on the Sci-Fi channel, along with *Battlestar Galactica*, in its 25th season.

What about the social justice movement in general? What does the famous Princeton honor code suggest might be honorable as you leave this haven? Don't we need an honor code that would honor this planet and all those living on it?

Of course we do, and here's another look at a utopian future.

By 2028, the war in Iraq will be long over, our troops *and* bases back home. Most vets will have gone to college; those who went with green cards will be citizens with access to health care just like everyone else. One of our nation's leaders, who will remain unnamed but who always looks grumpy and is not the best hunting companion, recently replied to the observation that most Americans opposed the war with a single word: "So?" But the administration following his will have found Americans' views more relevant to the shaping of our foreign policy and will have engaged in regional negotiations, under the aegis, heaven forefend, of the UN, to end the conflict in Iraq. The top twenty floors of the UN will still be there, and Halliburton stock, having slumped after the end of the war, will rise in value in 2020 because its primary activities will include supporting women's cooperatives throughout newly thriving African economies. The CEO of Halliburton will then be a Princeton-educated Rwandan woman shuttling between Kigali, Beijing, and the United States. When in Texas, she will speak fluent English and Spanish.

The country of Rwanda will not only have left poverty behind—eliminating malaria, cholera, and AIDS within its borders—but will have brokered peace in Sudan and offered development assistance to other countries in the region and, in two instances, in Europe. Rwandan businesswomen will have helped reconfigure a number of European businesses in order to keep them green, competitive, and focused not just on product but on those who produce. A new Darfur will host the summer Olympic games, having stopped, with the help of peacekeeping troops, the world's last genocide in 2009. China will have cut off support to the bad guys there, just as we Americans acknowledged a disturbing similarity to our unstinting support of medieval autocracies in the Middle East, also for access to oil and markets. Women in Saudi Arabia will have drivers' licenses and, at the same time, find it hard to retain a retinue of servants from the Philippines or Jordan, since those countries will be stable and affluent. In these regions, the men will help with the chores.

Nuclear proliferation will also have stopped. Einstein may or may not have believed in the afterlife, but somewhere, maybe in the ether over Palmer Hall, he will be smiling when in 2015 every country, including those on the by-then-defunct security council, began dismantling, really dismantling, their nuclear arsenals. The terms "cluster bomb" and "landmine" became dated but sometimes-colorful metaphors by the close of the second decade of the century.

By 2028, the decades-long trend of increasing social inequalities will have been reversed, and four of the world's five fast-est-growing economies will be in Africa. One of them will be Rwanda, with a GDP greater than Singapore's. Fair-trade coffee and tea will have given way to IT as Rwanda became, by 2020, the continent's high-tech leader.

Medicine and health care will have flourished during the first quarter of the twenty-first century. The United States will have a world-class national health system, introduced in 2009, with universal coverage implemented by 2012. Health care costs will have fallen even as average citizens live longer, better lives. "Social safety net" will no longer be a dirty word. In 2024, Shir-ley Tilghman will complete the Boston marathon in the senior division and, wearing bizarre orange spandex, become the first Ivy League president to do so in less than three hours. Harvard's longest-serving president, Drew Faust, will be right behind her, and that year, with all doping banned, cyclist and former Duke president Nan Keohane will win the Tour de France, senior division. This Gang of Three, as they'll be called, will have pushed the modern research university further along the path toward engagement with the world's poor, including those in this country.

There's the vision, Class of 2008. I would ask that the physi-cians present not pull out prescription pads to offer me anti-psy-chotic medications. How on earth could these wonderful devel-opments come to pass? Not through wishful thinking. But is it crazy to wish for these improvements? Is it crazy for the Class of 2008 to wish for something better than what has gone before? For hope and history to rhyme? Imagine a commencement speaker in the early nineteenth century, exhorting young Americans or Britons to abolish slavery as the affront to God that it surely was and is. Imagine an address in the early twentieth century in which the speaker pushed universal suffrage, arguing that an adult is an adult, regardless of race or gender. Imagine a speaker in 1993—not so long ago—arguing that apartheid in South Africa was an insult not just to the notion of human rights but to modernity itself. Imagine a country like ours looking back from 2028 and thinking it quaint that not that long ago a woman or a black would not likely be elected as our head of state. Imagine a world in which a global safety net makes work like mine easier, because we don't have to beg, borrow, and steal medicines and supplies after a natural disaster or after unfair trade rules wipe out food security in poor countries. A world in which every child has the right to go to school. A world in which clean water is not a privatized commodity to be sipped from bottles but rather part of the earth's bounty, for all its inhabitants.

For hope and history to rhyme, we need to build, or continue building, a social movement. To move forward any rights agenda, any plan for true progress, we must be part of a movement. We need to get on board.

Getting on board is a metaphor, of course. On board what, exactly? Like most of you here, I once lived in a bus. OK, so you didn't live on a bus, but for many years I lived with the other seven members of my family, not counting the dog, in a bus that had once been used in a tuberculosis-screening program in the city of Birmingham, Alabama. As tuberculosis became less of a threat to the public's health, the city and others sold off their mobile screening units in public bids. My father, ever alert to such events—he once bought a camo-colored car from the U.S. army for exactly $288—put in the winning bid on said bus. He promised us it was only for vacations, but before we knew it, we were living, all eight of us, in 28 feet of space.

I learned a lot, I now know, from living on the bus. I learned how to get along with my large, diverse family. And I learned, eventually, not to be embarrassed by the fact that we, unlike other families, did not live in a house or even a trailer. Yes, the bus taught me a lot.

I mention all this as a metaphor, of course, for the movement for environmental and social justice that you, Class of 2008, need to build. We all need to get on the bus and stay a while. For me, it's back on the bus, but no matter: it will be a great pleasure to be there with you, sitting in the rear as your generation steers through hard but better times.

That's my message to you all today. It's your job to drive that bus. It's your job to make hope and history rhyme. It's a heavy burden, but you can carry it: we know what happens to Princeton grads. You'll become scholars, scientists, physicians, lawyers, and titans of business. You'll become leaders in politics. Regardless of what it is you do during the next twenty years, you can be part of the movement to make life on this planet safer, more sustainable, and more just.

The inhabitants of our wounded but still wonderful world need you, Class of 2008. Make this long-hoped-for tidal wave wash away some of the world's problems, wash clean the wounds, and nourish the planet so that all of its inhabitants have a shot at the sort of marvelous lives that await you.

Congratulations and thank you, from the bottom of my orange heart, for inviting me here today. You inspire me more than you know.

The Drum Major Instinct

Boston University,
Martin Luther King Jr. Day Celebration

JANUARY 19, 2009

I. I HAVE A DREAM

Everybody knows Dr. Martin Luther King's four most famous words. They were spoken during his 1963 speech on the Mall in Washington. It's an event that is on a lot of people's minds these days because of another event that is shortly to take place in Washington and that might be taken to confirm the ability of majority Americans, after decades of being pushed, educated, and transformed, to judge each other "not . . . by the color of their skin but by the content of their character."

Today I've been invited to reflect on another of Dr. King's sermons, less well known than the "I have a dream" speech, but one with a message for this week and this moment in our country's history. I am honored to make these comments at Dr. King's alma mater on the day people across the world honor his memory. Although my remarks concern the worldwide struggle to reach our full promise as humans—with rights inalienable in principle but far from obtained—I will not be coy about their intended meaning for Americans on the eve of the inauguration of President Barack Obama.

It is fitting that this year's MLK celebration has blurred into our inauguration of a new president. I'll bet we'll hear references tomorrow not only to Lincoln but also to King. Both have much to teach us, both are part of that arc of history that bends, however slowly, toward justice. And as Lincoln's brooding marble image presides over the proceedings, so too will MLK's rhetoric of dreams suffuse our hearts, today and tomorrow.

The dream described in the 1963 speech on the National Mall was about equality. "The Drum Major Instinct," Dr. King's last sermon at Ebenezer Baptist Church, in 1968, is about leadership. Don't these two speeches seem to head in opposite directions: equality being for all of us, leadership a role only a few can play? But as Dr. King analyzes it, what he calls the "Drum Major Instinct" is the desire, probably innate in all of us, for the praise and recognition that come with leadership. Who doesn't fantasize about being in charge, whether as drum major in a marching band or as leader of a movement or head of a department or, even, as president of a flawed but promising democracy? These roles gratify our hunger for applause and approval. But King also saw the darker side of leadership. He spoke rawly and honestly about the dangers inherent in "keeping up with the Joneses" and of striving to impress through material advantage. In particular, he had his eye on the treacherous point where the quest for excellence and for personal efficacy compromises the broader goals of equality and justice for all.

Dr. King is now an American icon. But we can't forget that he was a controversial figure in his time—controversial even among his supporters, who couldn't always see where he was going or how the parts of his program fit together. If it was difficult for some people in 1968 to understand the complexity of King's reflections on theology or on the struggle of poor people in far-off Vietnam, it can't be so difficult for any of us to see how the greater good might be damaged by one person's overweening efforts to be the best, to lead. We recognize ourselves in the straw man of "The Drum Major Instinct." There's a reason, surely, that Coretta Scott King asked that this sermon be replayed at his funeral. For in this homily, Dr. King, Nobel laureate and hero to millions, refers presciently to his own funeral and asks that no mention of his many awards and honors be made. Let it only be said, he asked, that he strove to "feed the hungry," to "clothe the naked," to "be right on the [Vietnam] war question," and to "love and serve humanity."

To feed the hungry, clothe the naked, stand up for peace, and love and serve humanity—these issues, transcendent today, are central to the ideals any doctor might have regarding the right to health. They are precisely the priorities that should guide public policy and private action in times of economic turmoil. How do we accomplish these aims without making them serve our own love of glory and admiration? How do we, gathered here today, on January 19, 2009, at Boston University, fit into a plan larger than ourselves? What do all of us, with our potential for leading and for following, have to offer in a struggle that might move us beyond our own ineradicable Drum Major Instinct without dampening our desire to succeed?

If MLK were with us today, in flesh and not (as he is) in spirit, he would surely be pleased by the events that will unfold tomorrow in our nation's capital. But he would not regard this momentous event, the inauguration, as the end of the struggle, but as an opening, a chance, a space in which a much broader social justice agenda might be ushered in. In making this claim, I do not also claim to know King personally, though I did live in Birmingham for a time. I was eight years old when he was taken from us. But his speeches, sermons, and actions leave us with little doubt about his views on justice, views which would not be vindicated by Barack Obama's gaining high office unless that office were used to pursue a more just vision of our nation and our world. Likewise, there's little doubt about Dr. King's views on the wars conducted on the basis of lies: simply speaking out, even from a position of power, against such wars will not suffice.

If MLK had a dream toward the end of his life, it was the dream of more radical equity. It is for this reason that he has never faded away, as have many other noble people martyred for their just beliefs. MLK's mature dreams, those laid out with clarity in the last months of his life, are precisely those we need to inspire us in a time of great need.

II. DREAM OR NIGHTMARE?

In a celebration like this one and in a time like ours that is fraught with promise and peril, it's possible to forget the hard work still before all of us. In "Letter from Birmingham Jail," Dr. King famously noted that "we will have to repent in this generation not merely for the hateful words and actions of the bad people but for the appalling silence of the good people." Just as it was the silence of good people that permitted some of the excesses of recent years—for me these include not only the war in Iraq but also the overthrow, yet again, of democracy in Haiti and also our appalling silence on the right to health care in our own country—it is also the collective roar of good people that promises to redress them. Many of you will agree: we are even today filling appalling silences with a loud and optimistic chorus of commitment to doing better. Certainly, I hear the loud roar of the students!

We know, of course, that good intentions are not sufficient to do the job, any more than is reluctant compliance with progress. After leaving the tumult of Alabama shortly after King's death, I still remember waiting with my five brothers and sisters for the school bus in a small Florida town. Jim Crow had been struck down legally, but at the gas station that served as our bus stop were two bathrooms. They were labeled "Men" and "Women," but above these labels were, still readable, the ghostly shadows of other words announcing different criteria for entry, which had been painted over not long before. The image sticks in my mind as much as the grainy, black-and-white photographs of MLK in DC.

The stain of Jim Crow, itself the legacy of slavery, will, like the fates meted out to Native Americans, be with us always. But what is the message in such dramatic changes as we have seen since MLK made the ultimate sacrifice? Or even since 1992, when the theologian James Cone wrote a book called *Martin & Malcolm & America: A Dream or a Nightmare?* In it, Cone asked not so much how far we've come but rather how the visions of MLK and Malcolm X came together toward the end. Both were fighting, in their own ways, for a vision of social justice. MLK embraced a Gandhian perspective on this struggle and was criticized for it by some in the movement. In many ways, he has been vindicated. Malcolm was less ready to limit the struggle to non-violent resistance, and his legacy has been more mixed. But it would be incorrect to deny him credit as a force for justice and social change.

The ghost of white supremacy continues to fade, here as elsewhere. The difference between the conditions that brought MLK to the Mall in the sixties and those that will bring Barack

Obama to the Mall tomorrow is patent and deserves to be celebrated—and we should do so on both of these days. But the
all-encompassing struggle for social justice is in some ways in its
infancy. MLK understood this, especially toward the end of his
life, as clearly as anyone.

III. HUMAN RIGHTS AND SOCIAL JUSTICE

In some ways, King has become like other iconic leaders, a
screen against which we project our hopes and aspirations. The
same can be said about our president-elect, and that's a heavy
burden to carry. Let's take King, not as an icon, but as a work in
progress. Take him in those years between 1963 and 1968. He was
moving forward on his own intellectual and moral and political path. After all, there was MLK the seminarian, MLK the
doctoral student at BU, MLK the preacher, MLK the national
leader, MLK the Nobel laureate, and MLK of the poor people's
movement. He was, as they say, all that. He knew what he was
talking about when he warned against the Drum Major Instinct.
He was changing and growing and learning all the time—and
guarding against any tendency in himself to take credit, to take
charge, to treat a social movement as his personal accessory.

   In celebrating Dr. King, we need to respect his own trajectory and growth, not just the final form of his name, the post-
age stamps, monuments, chapters in history books. We need to
acknowledge that he was working toward a goal: the fight for
social justice for all, the fight against poverty. "The curse of
poverty has no justification in our age," he wrote in 1967. "The
time has come for us to civilize ourselves by the total, direct and
immediate abolition of poverty."[21]

   As in his final sermon, he spoke of the hungry, the naked,

the homeless, the thirsty, the vulnerable. Elsewhere, he spoke explicitly of health disparities, and in a way that no doctor should fail to appreciate. "Of all the forms of inequality," he said, "injustice in health care is the most shocking and inhumane."[22] Will this form of inequality be addressed in our lifetimes?

And he took on the great controversies of the day. Here's what he said about the Vietnam War: "The bombs in Vietnam explode at home; they destroy the hopes and possibilities for a decent America."[23] He opposed the war for several reasons, but perhaps the most important ones were that he regarded the justification for the war as fraudulent:

> We are adding cynicism to the process of death, for they [U.S. troops in Vietnam] must know after a short period there that none of the things we claim to be fighting for are really involved. Before long they must know that their government has sent them into a struggle among Vietnamese, and the more sophisticated surely realize that we are on the side of the wealthy and the secure while we create a hell for the poor.[24]

MLK also believed the resources spent on war should be spent on the war on poverty. He argued that "a nation that continues year after year to spend more money on military defense than on programs of social uplift is approaching spiritual death."[25] In expressing these views, King was not seeking to win a popularity contest. A significant fraction of the mainstream media—journals that had previously praised King—voiced their opposition to his opposition. *Life* magazine termed the speech in which these words were uttered "demagogic slander that sounded like a script for Radio Hanoi."[26] The *Washington Post* opined that he had "diminished his usefulness to his cause, his country, his people."[27] The Drum Major Instinct, if not held in check, might well have led King to accept postures more palatable to the mainstream media, the newspapers, magazines, and television programs that had celebrated him in previous years.

Here's what he said about hunger: "I started thinking about the fact that we spend millions of dollars a day to store surplus food in our country. And I said to myself, 'I know where we can store that food free of charge: in the wrinkled stomachs of the millions of God's children in Asia and Africa, in South America, and in our own nation, who go to bed hungry tonight.'"[28]

This is not ancient history. Don't we still need to deplore unjust wars today? The bombing of civilian populations? Don't we still need to think about social justice? About hunger that causes food riots in cities across the globe? Don't we need, in the midst of financial crisis, to reflect on King's argument that "true compassion is more than flinging a coin to a beggar. . . . [True compassion] comes to see that an edifice which produces beggars needs restructuring"?[29]

IV. ACCEPTING OUR NEED TO CELEBRATE

It would be possible to end these remarks in a scolding or otherwise negative tone. I might have reminded all of you that Dr. King was willing to die for his convictions, did not shrink from danger, and faced death bravely and calmly. I might have insisted that because we still confront injustice—even racial injustice—we have made too little progress. I might have underlined only what is wrong and failed to signal what it right and promising and new.

I do not choose to do that today.

Today we celebrate the life and legacy of Martin Luther King. Today we celebrate his courage and his paradoxical relationship to the Drum Major Instinct. Without that instinct, he would not have pursued either his career or his vocation. Had he lacked it, he would not have gone to jail, nor would he have spoken to millions, directly and with courage. But Dr. King was aware of the risks of seeking to elevate himself above others, and it is for this reason, among others, that he sought to ground himself in the struggles of the poor in this country and elsewhere. It is for this reason that he never became a "brand," to use the language of our day.

Let us all take inspiration from a man who, years after receiving a Nobel Prize, would seek to learn and to grow, a man willing to take on conventional wisdom, even when it rankled some of his supporters and many of his fair-weather friends. Let us celebrate the optimism of MLK. He never failed to believe in the promise of our species. Fallible humanity was his inspiration every bit as much as his God. Redemption is always possible. "We must accept finite disappointment," he cautioned, "but never lose infinite hope."[30]

Finally, we need to learn to acknowledge and harness the Drum Major Instinct within all of us, the urge to be somebody and to succeed. If not for that impulse, who among us would be here today, at one of the great universities of this country? I know I would not be here as a physician and teacher. Barack Obama would not be our nation's 44th president. But the greatest thing about King's redemptive vision is that all of us may, at any time, choose to place the well-being of others above our own. All of us may strive for compassion, justice, and altruism. None of us need have the vision, talent, and heroism of an MLK to succeed in this humble and necessary task. "Everybody can be great," said Dr. King, "because anybody can serve."[31]

Now—as our country and our world faces financial crisis, environmental disaster, war, and growing inequality—is a time to serve. It's a time to concern ourselves with the oppressed or those less fortunate. It's a time to do what many BU students have done: to draw on deep reserves of compassion and solidarity and, above all, to engage in the movement to make the world safer, more just, more humane. If this is what we do with our Drum Major Instinct, we need not be troubled by it.

Everybody can be great, because anybody can serve.

Thank you all.

Accompaniment as Policy

Harvard Kennedy School of Government,
Commencement

MAY 25, 2011

Rudolf Virchow, one of the heroes of public health, contended that "medicine is a social science, and politics is nothing other than medicine writ large."[32] That was in 1848, and it would please me greatly to think that Virchow's point has been taken. In any case, I'm grateful for the invitation to deliver a commencement address at the Kennedy School, where governance and policy are the focus of your studies.

Although I'm a physician, these past two years have been an object lesson about the difficulties of scaling up—of moving from caring for individual patients to building health systems in settings of privation and disarray. A few years ago, building health systems was precisely the arena I thought I knew most about. But the January 2010 earthquake that ended so many Haitian lives and destroyed so much of Port-au-Prince was a grim

An abridged version of this speech was published online by Foreign Affairs. See "Partners in Help: Assisting the Poor over the Long Term," *Foreign Affairs* July 29, 2011, http://www.foreignaffairs.com/articles/68002/paul-farmer/part ners-in-help.

reminder that we still lack the ability to translate goodwill and resources into robust responses to disasters natural and unnatural. Today I will reflect mostly on lessons learned in Haiti. But I believe that the lessons carry over to far less dramatically disrupted settings, including this city and this country, and I invite you to reflect with me on the present state—the limits and the potential—of the activity that used to be called charity or foreign aid. I hope to convince you all this morning that we should move *from aid to accompaniment.*

I.

"Accompaniment" is an elastic term. It has a basic, everyday meaning. To accompany someone is to go somewhere with him or her, to break bread together, to be present on a journey with a beginning and an end. There's an element of mystery, of openness, of trust, in accompaniment. The companion, the accompagnateur, says: "I'll go with you and support you on your journey wherever it leads. I'll share your fate for a while"—and by "a while," I don't mean a little while. Accompaniment is about sticking with a task until it's deemed completed—not by the accompagnateur, but by the person being accompanied.

I teach here at Harvard but volunteer with Partners In Health, an organization I helped to found over 25 years ago. We've sought to make accompaniment the cornerstone of our efforts, from rural Haiti to the prisons of Siberia to the hard-up neighborhoods of Boston. In every setting in which we've worked, there are people who need accompaniment: patients with chronic disease, families facing loss or chronic troubles (most linked to poverty, such as insufficient food or shelter), but also health officials and doctors and nurses who lack ready access to the tools of our trade. In other words, even the erstwhile accompagnateurs need accompaniment. The concept is not diluted by noting that everyone who draws breath needs accompaniment at some stage of life, as long as we acknowledge that some need it more than others.

There's no one-size-fits-all approach to accompaniment, but there are surely some basic principles. I first heard the term "accompagnateur"—the Haitian word for someone who accompanies—in 1982. It was the year following my graduation from college, and I found myself in Cange, a squatter settlement in central Haiti. I've told this story many times, to my own students and to anyone who'll listen, but hope it bears repeating today. Why were those people gathered in rickety thatch huts on a dusty hilltop? Because they'd been displaced by a "development" project, a hydroelectric dam that flooded a fertile valley in order to improve agribusiness downstream and to send electricity to far-off Port-au-Prince. (The dam was built by a company later absorbed by a tiny concern named Halliburton.) Irrigation and electrification are worthy goals. But the people I was living among blamed their misfortune on an infrastructure project that was, at the time of its completion, one of the largest buttress dams in the world, located in one of the poorest countries in the world.

In 1984, as a first-year medical student, I returned to Haiti often to work with community health workers; we had not yet recruited doctors or nurses since we had not yet completed the clinic we were building in Cange. When community health workers confronted acute illness in their home villages, they began referring patients to the nascent clinic, which a decade later became a small hospital and then, still later, a medical center. But we learned early on that patients with chronic disease, from tuberculosis to diabetes, needed a lot more than the momentary medical attention one receives at a clinical facility: they needed long-term social support.

The families we sought to serve lived in deep poverty. Without food and clean water and adequate housing, they would not fully benefit from medical care. So we adjusted our approach, making financial and nutritional support central to our tuberculosis program, and training community health workers to deliver care to afflicted neighbors. These changes boosted cure rates as much as they did morale. Simply getting from their villages to the clinic was a challenge for our patients, who needed help with transportation and child care. You may have missed our paper in *Seminars in Respiratory Infections* twenty years ago, but I believe it introduced the term "donkey-rental fee" to the medical literature.[33]

We took to calling such complex wraparound services *accompaniment.* Community health workers were more than distributors of medicine and keepers of records; they were patients' accompagnateurs. And we found that when good clinical care—the right diagnosis and treatment plan—is followed by robust accompaniment, we could expect cure rates for tuberculosis to go from around 50 percent to closer to 100 percent.[34] When HIV reached these villages, at the close of the eighties, we accompanied people living with AIDS.

Our teams brought this same strategy to Roxbury, Dorchester, Mattapan, and other poorer neighborhoods in and around Boston. People living in the shadows of Harvard's great teaching hospitals—suffering from chronic and incurable diseases while also suffering from chronic and sometimes curable poverty—needed medical accompaniment in their homes and communities if they were to stay on schedule with appointments and meds. They also had trouble finding child care and keeping up on rent, and accompaniment that addressed these difficulties improved their clinical prognoses.[35]

II.

So far, I've described a couple of small *programs* that brought modern health care to those who happened to live in the regions in which we worked. But after years of hard work, we looked around us and saw that we still lived in a world where many millions died each year of treatable infectious diseases. Medicine and wraparound services could do only so much. It was ultimately a series of *policy* decisions that infused new resources into the diagnosis and care of chronic illnesses, including AIDS and tuberculosis, in some of the poorest parts of the world. Some of these ideas were first discussed here at the Kennedy School with the economist Jeffrey Sachs, who invited me to address a class here in the late 1990s. I returned the favor by inviting Sachs to visit my mainstay squatter settlement in Haiti.

Sachs and his wife, Sonia, a pediatrician, had come to see our "controversial" AIDS program. Why might it be controversial to treat AIDS in "resource-poor settings"? The answer: because of a failure of imagination. The drugs were deemed too costly for poor people. *Newsweek* even printed a cover with the image of a young man dying from AIDS with the title "Too Poor to Treat," and mass outrage, as far as I know, did not erupt.[36] Despite this consensus of indifference, Jeffrey Sachs, who as an economist should have a good idea about what things cost, decided to come to Cange and see for himself. Now of course, Cange looked different in 2000 than it had in 1983: the dust had been replaced by trees and green; there were schools and a hospital; lean-tos had been replaced by tin-roofed homes. It was far from perfect, but it was immeasurably better than two decades previously.

Sachs wasn't feeling well during that visit, and I, responsible doctor that I am, suggested that a brisk walk to a village about two hours away would do him good. I almost killed Jeffrey Sachs. Five hours in the blazing sun did not, in fact, improve Professor Sachs's clinical status.

Nonetheless, he did get to see community health workers—accompagnateurs—tending to patients with AIDS. These patients were doing just fine, now that they had access to the fruits of modern medicine.[37] This was significant in ways that transcended the specific challenges facing Haiti because AIDS had become, by then, the world's leading infectious killer of young adults.

But there was no available funding to link HIV prevention to proper care on a large scale. The history of the rise in funding over the past decade has yet to be written fully, but the Global Fund to Fight AIDS, Tuberculosis and Malaria, a financing mechanism proposed by Sachs that took shape in 2002, was one milestone on the road to countering unnecessary suffering and death. The U.S. President's Emergency Plan for AIDS Relief (PEPFAR), launched the following year, was another. These efforts have saved millions of lives, mostly young lives, over the past years.

The Global Fund and PEPFAR also set a precedent for life-long accompaniment of people living in poverty and facing incurable but treatable diseases. They raised the bar in global health. Although these initiatives targeted AIDS, tuberculosis, and malaria, think also about diabetes or mental illness or cancer, which are great and chronic scourges in settings of poverty. Might similar funds become available to fight these diseases?

What about the "neglected tropical diseases," so named because they attract little attention despite being significant causes of global mortality and morbidity? The list goes on and on. We hope the Global Fund, PEPFAR, and other initiatives launched in the last decade may usher in a more ambitious era in the history of global health. We also hope that health care reform in the United States will lead to home-based accompaniment for chronic disease and to increased support for community health workers in this country.

III.

Accompaniment is an elastic term, but not too elastic. It is not the same as a paid consultancy or a one-off project to help certain institutions or individuals for a time. As noted, the beginning of accompaniment is often clearer than the end. There is a theological literature on accompaniment, and if you have the temerity to plumb it, you will be reminded of the term's Latin origins: *ad* + *cum* + *panis*, one way of saying "breaking bread together."[38]

The term crops up especially in liberation theology, which has its roots in Latin America, where Partners In Health also has its deepest roots. PIH is a secular organization, but many of us draw on inspiring work by people like Gustavo Gutiérrez, a Peruvian priest who has written compellingly of "the preferential option for the poor."[39]

This became a guiding principle of our work: although everyone deserves decent medical care, those living in poverty receive the lion's share of our attention. As any epidemiologist can tell you, diseases themselves make a grim and preferential choice to strike the poor. Our life's work would be to accompany the destitute sick on a journey away from premature suffering and death.

Of course these two notions—an option for the poor and accompaniment—are linked. In a book about a theology of accompaniment, Roberto Goizueta writes, "To 'opt for the poor' is thus to place ourselves *there*, to *accompany* the poor person in his or her life, death, and struggle for survival."[40] Professor Goizueta, who draws heavily on the work of Father Gutiérrez, is focused on the accompaniment of Latinos in this country. He writes about the importance of physical proximity to accompaniment:

> As a society, we are happy to help and serve the poor, as long as we don't have to walk *with* them where they walk, that is, as long as we can minister to them from our safe enclosures. The poor can then remain passive objects of our actions, rather than friends, *compañeros* and *compañeras*, with whom we interact. As long as we can be sure that we will not have to live with them, and thus have interpersonal relationships with them … we will try to help "the poor"—but, again, only from a controllable, geographical distance.[41]

IV.

So what might notions like accompaniment or a preferential option for the poor have to do with governance and enlightened policy? Let me draw on my experience responding to the earthquake that leveled much of Haiti's capital city a year and a half ago to compare conventional "aid" to what an accompaniment approach might look like.

After the quake, many countries and organizations offered to supply humanitarian assistance, and one of the jobs of the United Nations Office of the Special Envoy for Haiti, headed by President Clinton, was to track aid pledges for relief and reconstruction. Here are some startling numbers, especially if you're interested in strengthening public health and public education:

of the $2.4 billion committed or disbursed in the sixteen months after the quake, 34 percent was provided to civil and military entities of donor states; 30 percent was provided to UN agencies and international NGOs; 29 percent was provided to other NGOs and private contractors; 6 percent was provided in-kind to unspecified recipients; and 1 percent was provided to the Haitian government.[42]

A couple of caveats: first, these amounts were for humanitarian relief, not reconstruction. Second, it's hard to move resources through a government in ruins: 28 of 29 Haitian federal buildings were damaged or destroyed, and perhaps 20 percent of federal employees were killed or injured in the quake.[43] And God knows we needed the logistic and medical support of outfits like the USNS *Comfort*, which steamed into Haitian waters on day eight after the quake. But surely more could have been done to accompany local authorities who sought help in the business of relief and recovery. An accompaniment approach would require new rules of the road for foreign assistance.

If almost none of the direct relief money has gone to Haitian authorities, and very few of the reconstruction contracts are going to Haitian firms, where is all this aid going?[44] A lot of it goes to foreign contractors and international NGOs, which often have high overheads. Some of you graduating today will soon be leading such organizations, if you don't already, and you will need to help find a better way of accompanying our development partners.

Local job creation is a hallmark of an accompaniment approach. Sometimes this will include more direct budgetary support for struggling public health and education authorities, more support for local firms, and more local procurement. Of course, competition for resources—jobs, lucrative contracts, and the like—can provoke discord. But certain projects, including medical care for the poorest and education of the young, should be supported by a broad consensus.

An example: one of the lessons we've learned since the early days is that it's difficult, sometimes impossible, to treat patients who don't get enough food to eat. As many as half of school-aged children in Haiti, and almost all those we meet in clinics and hospitals, live with chronic "food insecurity," to use the jargon of the day. One remedy for acute malnutrition is known as ready-to-use therapeutic food—RUTF for short. Colleagues from Médecins Sans Frontières showed in Niger that a miraculous and tasty peanut paste could save the lives of most children with moderate and acute malnutrition.[45] For years, we've used a similar recipe in central Haiti to make what we call *Nourimanba*. (*Manba* is the Haitian word for peanut butter.) Instead of buying this paste from abroad, we made our own using mostly locally procured ingredients—an obvious choice in a predominantly agricultural country like Haiti. After starting in the pharmacy warehouse in Cange, we soon built a tiny production facility. As in Niger, we found the miracle paste worked well in treating moderate and severe malnutrition. The reliable market for peanuts created by this endeavor also helped lessen the food insecurity of local farmers.

We're now working on a larger-scale facility with improved food-processing capacity. Although this effort has demanded skills beyond our team's medical training, we found many partners, including Haitian agronomists and specialists from a U.S. pharmaceutical company. This effort will not only treat all children diagnosed with acute malnutrition in our clinics, but also provide many jobs and use, whenever possible, locally procured ingredients. It ends up, therefore, being accompaniment not only for malnourished children and their families, but also for local farmers and all those seeking to improve food-processing capacity in rural Haiti.

It would have been easier perhaps to buy RUTF on the international marketplace. If the ingredients were difficult to obtain or prepare, as is the case with many vaccines, ordering from abroad might have been the only alternative. But RUTF seems a good example of a product that can and should be prepared locally.[46]

Another example: Port-au-Prince's general hospital is charged with the largest patient load in the city, but it has too few resources and medical personnel. Its staff was small and underpaid even before the quake. In the weeks and months after January 12, many international teams set up shop on the general hospital campus, helping to bolster its surgical capacity and acute care, and also to keep track of patients. Coordination was a challenge: different relief groups sometimes vied for space or control over hospital facilities. But no one could deny the essential part played by rescue and relief teams in mitigating a great deal of suffering and death in the quake's aftermath.

When many disaster relief teams packed their bags, however, the hospital was still overrun with patients requiring medical attention; its staff was still underpaid. Our teams have tried to bring together a number of international partners interested in traveling the longer and harder road of recovery and reconstruction—in this case, helping rebuild the general hospital. The American Red Cross agreed to send $3.8 million in "performance-based" salary support for the hospital's beleaguered employees. This work has been difficult and slow: Haitian institutions often lack the infrastructure of transparency and platforms for evaluation (electricity, modern bookkeeping, accountants, computers) demanded by most donors' account-ability norms. But only an accompaniment approach will help develop such platforms and put them under the control of the intended beneficiaries. The Red Cross collaboration is starting to bear fruit: the staff is better paid; accountability platforms are taking root.

We've come to believe that this kind of accompaniment—partnering with Haitian institutions and working through what-ever obstacles present themselves—is among the best ways to help address the structural deficits preventing Haiti from rebuilding better.[47]

v.

I have been talking about accompaniment as an objective set at the beginning of a task and as a mode of follow-through. My intended lesson, in a nutshell, is this: the great failures of policy and governance usually occur because of *failures of implementation,* and *accompaniment* is good insurance against such failures.

There are, of course, many bad policies; they've scarred the world in diverse ways and damage the vulnerable most of all. But most policies cooked up in places like the Kennedy School are not bad policies. Most policies developed by UN agencies or Ministries of Health are not bad policies. When NGOs take the trouble to develop policies, which isn't all that often, they are also not bad policies. The problem is delivery.

When Corail-Cesselesse, a windswept plain north of Port-au-Prince, was identified as a possible post-earthquake reset-tlement location, scores of architects and urban planners set to work developing plans by the dozens. But months dragged on, and still no one had broken ground. In fact, no one even bothered to check whether the proposed site was suitable for implementation. The tendency to "minister from safe enclosures," to use Professor Goizueta's words, rather than from the place itself led planners to overlook the minor detail that Corail sat smack in the middle of a floodplain. Anything built there would have sunk in the mud during the rainy season.

Of course, *failures of imagination* are the really costly failures. Malcolm Gladwell quotes an engineer speaking of his former employer: "Xerox had been infested by a bunch of spreadsheet experts who thought you could decide every project based on metrics. Unfortunately, creativity wasn't on a metric."[48] Neither are goodness or decency or social justice or accompaniment. But that doesn't mean we don't need these traits in public policy and in service of the common good. Just because we cannot yet measure the value of accompaniment doesn't mean it cannot serve as a guiding principle.

Another way of putting this is "Beware the iron cage." About 25 years ago, when I was a graduate student here in two different fields, medicine and anthropology, I went to the Coop to buy an enormous book by the sociologist Max Weber. It hurt my back and brain to even look at this giant tome, but his topic—how the "iron cage" of rationality comes to suppress individual agency and innovation—remains relevant to this day. This occurs by "routinization," the process in which rationalized bureaucracies gradually assume power in modern society. This is often a good thing: rationalized procedures can improve efficiency and equity. Atul Gawande has made this insight the core of his "Checklist Manifesto."[49] When the World Health Organization launched its directly observed therapy short-course (DOTS) protocol for tuberculosis—as noted, the notion of directly observed care is, in some sense, an outgrowth of accompaniment—many countries (like Peru) made great strides toward controlling TB, a scourge that had been around for centuries.

But this form of efficiency runs up against its limits when exceptional events—"black swans"—appear. When patients began falling ill to drug-resistant strains of TB, DOTS guidelines suggested they be treated with the same first-line drugs used in the existing protocol. Giving patients the very drugs to which their TB had developed resistance not only failed to help them, it enabled resistant strains to spread unchecked, often first among the patients' families and coworkers (if these patients had jobs).[50] This example demonstrates the double-edged sword of routinization: the rationalized protocols of DOTS first helped health providers increase the effectiveness and reach of TB treatment but later blinded them to steps necessary to curb the spread of emerging drug-resistant strains. Increases in bureaucratic efficiency come at the price of decreasing the ability of human actors to be flexible, to respond to problems creatively and promptly. In other words, as institutions are rationalized, and as platforms of accountability are strengthened, the potential for accompaniment can be threatened, since it is, as noted, open-ended, egalitarian, elastic, and nimble.

When the iron cage of rationality leads to an imaginative poverty, cynicism and disengagement follow.[51] It's easy to be dismissive of accompaniment in a world in which technical expertise is advanced as the answer to every problem. But expertise alone will not solve the difficult problems. This was the long, hard lesson of the earthquake: we all waited to be saved by expertise, and it never came. Accompaniment does not privilege technical prowess above solidarity or compassion or a willingness to tackle what may seem to be insuperable challenges. It requires cooperation, openness, and teamwork of the sort so many of you cherish. Much more can be accomplished, looking forward, with an open-source view of the world. Ideas for good governance, whether of organizations or government bureaucracies or corporations, are meant to be shared and shared widely. This is true of sectors public and private.[52]

You were admitted to the Kennedy School because you were already leaders, already accomplished, and deemed likely to make an even greater difference with skills, knowledge, and ideas garnered here. I have no doubt that you will go forth and lead thoughtfully. May the idea of accompaniment go with you on your own journeys, wherever they take you.

Godspeed and thank you all.

NOTES

INTRODUCTION

1. Many of his academic writings are collected in *Partner to the Poor: A Paul Farmer Reader* (Berkeley: University of California Press, 2010).

2. The course is currently in its fifth year and continues to attract hundreds of students each term it is offered. An introductory global health textbook, which was modeled on this course, is forthcoming. *Reimagining Global Health: An Introduction* (Berkeley: University of California Press, in press).

3. For more on this topic, see Paul's book *Infections and Inequalities: The Modern Plagues* (University of California Press, 1999).

4. E. Marseille, P. Hofmann, and J. Kahn, "HIV Prevention before HAART in Sub-Saharan Africa," *The Lancet* 359, no. 9320 (May 25, 2002): 1851–56.

5. Myron Cohen et al., "Prevention of HIV-1 Infection with Early Antiretroviral Therapy," *The New England Journal of Medicine* 11, no. 365 (August 2011): 493–505.

6. UNAIDS, "2012 World AIDS Day Report—Results," (2012), http://www.unaids.org/en/resources/documents/2012/.

7. Henry David Thoreau, *Walden* (New York: Thomas Y. Crowell and Co., 1910), 47.

8. Vaccination is an imperfect tool, and an expanded vaccine effort must not undermine the treatment of patients and the provision of clean water and modern sanitation. Strong public-sector water and sanitation systems would halt transmission of cholera and also that of other waterborne pathogens, such as typhoid fever and hepatitis A, which also claim many lives among the poor, especially among children. Paul and I wrote a longer piece exploring some of the claims of causality about cholera control in Haiti and elsewhere in *Americas Quarterly*, http://americasquarterly.org/cholera-and-the-road-to-modernity.

9. See also Arthur Kleinman's work on the moral dimensions of caregiving, for example: "Caregiving: The Odyssey of Becoming More Human," *The Lancet* 373, no. 9660 (2009): 292–93.

10. See, for example: J. W. Carlson et al., "Partners in Pathology: A Collaborative Model to Bring Pathology to Resource Poor Settings," *American Journal of Surgery and Pathology* 34, no.1 (2010): 118–23; Carole Mitnick et al., "Community-based Therapy for Multidrug-resistant Tuberculosis in Lima, Peru," *New England Journal of Medicine* 348, no. 2 (2003): 119–22; P. Farmer et al., "Community-based Approaches to HIV Treatment in Resource-poor Settings," *The Lancet* 358 (2001): 404–409; Giuseppe Raviola et al., "Mental Health Response in Haiti in the Aftermath of the 2010 Earthquake: A Case Study for Building Long-term Solutions," *Harvard Review of Psychiatry* 20, no. 201 (2012): 68–77.

11. Paul Farmer, "Accompaniment as Policy," Kennedy School of Government Commencement Speech 2011, in this volume.

12. For example, many donors favor so-called vertical programs that target specific diseases. While such efforts can make inroads against major causes of mortality and morbidity, they reflect priorities cooked up in boardrooms in Washington or Geneva, not necessarily the priorities of the poor. By adopting an accompaniment approach, PIH learned that initiatives to combat leading killers such as AIDS and tuberculosis could be improved by providing primary health care and "wraparound" social and economic services, such as food support or improved housing. Strengthening health systems is a taller task than tackling a single disease but one that surely brings greater long-term

return on investment in terms of stemming death and disability, not to mention generating beneficial spillover effects on local economies.

13. Paul Farmer, "Countering Failures of Imagination," Northwestern University Commencement Speech 2012, in this volume.

PART I: REIMAGINING EQUITY

1. I have the late philosopher Richard Rorty's word on this. See Richard Rorty, "The Communitarian Impulse," speech given at Colorado College's 125th Anniversary Symposium, Cultures in the 21st Century: Conflicts and Convergences, Colorado Springs, CO (February 5, 1999).

2. Drew Faust, *This Republic of Suffering: Death and the American Civil War* (New York: Vintage Books, 2008).

3. This is the thesis, at any rate, of the forthcoming textbook that might be considered a sort of companion volume to this one. See Paul Farmer et al., *Reimagining Global Health: An Introduction* (Berkeley: University of California Press, in press).

4. As Paul Wise observes, "Too often, those who elevate the role of social determinants [of health] indict clinical technologies as failed strategies. But devaluing clinical intervention diverts attention from the essential goal that it be provided equitably to all those in need. Belittling the role of clinical care tends to unburden policy of the requirement to provide equitable access to such care." See "Confronting Racial Disparities in Infant Mortality: Reconciling Science and Politics," *American Journal of Preventive Medicine* 9, no. 6 (1993): 9.

5. MEDLINE contains journal citations and abstracts for biomedical literature from around the world.

6. P.G. Wodehouse, *Right Ho, Jeeves* (Rockville, Maryland: Arc Manor Books), 145.

7. Plato, *Republic*, Book 1, 341-C.

8. Joseph Kahn, "Rich Nations Consider Fund of Billions to Fight AIDS," the *New York Times*: April 29, 2001, http://www.nytimes.com/2001/04/29/world/rich-nations-consider-fund-of-billions-to-fight-aids.html.

9. The Krebs' Cycle, also known as the citric acid cycle, is a sequence of chemical reactions that are a fundamental part of cellular metabolism.

10. D. V. Exner et al., "Lesser Response to Angiotensin-Converting-Enzyme Inhibitor Therapy in Black as Compared with White Patients with Left Ventricular Dysfunction," *New England Journal of Medicine* 344 (2001): 1351–57; R.S. Schwarz, "Racial Profiling in Medical Research," *New England Journal of Medicine* 344, no. 18 (2001): 1392–93.

11. Peter Schworm, "For Sendoff, Grads Prefer Big Name," *Boston Globe,* May 12, 2005, http://www.boston.com/news/local/articles/2005/05/12/for_sendoff_grads_prefer_big_names?pg=full.

12. Father William P. Leahy, a historian of religion and education in the United States, has served as president of Boston College since 1996.

13. The "peculiar institution" was a euphemism for slavery in the United States. See, for example, John C Calhoun's "Speech on the Reception of Abolition Petitions," Feb 6, 1837, http://users.wfu.edu/zulick/340/calhoun2.html.

14. Adam Hochschild, *Bury the Chains: Prophets and Rebels in the Fight to Free an Empire's Slaves* (New York: Houghton Mifflin, 2005), 89.

15. Hochschild, 89.

16. Hochschild, 90.

17. Pedro Arrupe, S.J., "Men for Others," address given to the Tenth International Congress of Jesuit Alumni of Europe, Valencia, Spain (July 31, 1973).

18. Roméo Dallaire, *Shake Hands with the Devil: The Failure of Humanity in Rwanda* (New York, Carroll & Graf Publishers, 2003).

19. Dallaire, 322.

20. Joseph Stiglitz and Linda Bilmes, *The Three Trillion Dollar War: The True Cost of the Iraq Conflict* (New York: W. W. Norton & Company, 2008).

21. This speech was given at the 2008 Skoll World Forum, an annual gathering of social entrepreneurs. The mission statement of the Skoll Foundation reads as follows: "to drive large scale change by investing in, connecting and celebrating social entrepreneurs and the innova-

tors who help them solve the world's most pressing problems," (http://www.skollfoundation.org/about).

22. The Skoll Foundation was launched by Jeff Skoll in 1999 and has been headed up by Sally Osberg since 2001.

23. International Campaign to Ban Landmines, *Landmine Monitor Report 1999: Toward a Mine-Free World* (1999); Human Rights Watch, "Exposing the Source: U.S. Companies and the Production of Antipersonnel Mines," *Human Rights Watch Arms Project* 9, no. 2 (1997); UNICEF, "Saving Children from the Tragedy of Landmines," Press Release, April 4, 2006.

24. For more on this story, see Paul Farmer, "'Landmine Boy' and the Tomorrow of Violence," in: B. Rylko-Bauer, L. Whiteford, and Paul Farmer, eds, *Global Health in Times of Violence* (Santa Fe, NM: SAR Press, 2009), 41–62.

25. See fig. 11 for photos of John before and after treatment.

26. Bertolt Brecht, "The World's One Hope," in *Poems 1913–1956* (London: Eyre Methuen, 1976), 328.

27. Paul Hawken, *Blessed Unrest: How the Largest Social Movement in History is Restoring Grace, Justice, and Beauty to the World* (London, UK: Penguin, 2008), 190.

28. Father Michael McFarland, a computer scientist and engineer, served as Holy Cross's president from 2000 to 2012.

29. These are the two mottos of Holy Cross.

30. Nicholas Lemann, "Evening the Odds: Is There a Politics of Inequality?" *New Yorker*, April 23, 2012.

31. Credit Suisse Research Institute, *Global Wealth Report* (October 2010).

32. John Maynard Keynes, "The Economic Possibilities of Our Grandchildren," in *Essays in Persuasion* (New York: Norton, 1963), 358–73.

33. Northwestern's 2012 honorary degree recipients included Martha Minow, Dean of Harvard Law School and renowned scholar of human rights law; William D. Nix, emeritus professor of engineering at Stanford University and a pioneering researcher in the mechanical properties of materials; and Joan Ganz Cooney, founder of Chil-

dren's Television Workshop (best known for its flagship program *Sesame Street*).

34. Morton Schapiro, an economist of higher education, has served as president of Northwestern University since 2009.

35. "The Rock" is a Northwestern campus landmark. "Painting the rock" is a tradition in which students cover the rock with images and slogans to draw attention to various causes and events. "Dillo Day" is Northwestern's biggest party. In 1972, a group of students organized a small party in honor of the armadillo, which over time evolved into an annual all-day music festival on the campus's lake fill.

PART II: THE FUTURE OF MEDICINE AND THE BIG PICTURE

1. Practitioners and scholars trained in anthropology, sociology, history, and epidemiology echo this critique. But none of these fields individually captures the biosocial complexity of health and illness in the world today; nor do they capture what Arthur Kleinman calls "the local moral worlds" of the patients and their families. See Arthur Kleinman and Joan Kleinman, "The Appeal of Experience; The Dismay of Images: Cultural Appropriations of Suffering in Our Times," in *Social Suffering*, ed. Arthur Kleinman et al. (Berkeley: University of California Press, 1997), 1–24. See also Arthur Kleinman, *What Really Matters: Living a Moral Life amidst Uncertainty and Danger* (Oxford: Oxford University Press, 2006).

2. Kleinman is now completing a book on the subject, which has loomed for him as much as spouse—he nursed his wife through a long and painful progressive illness—as physician. See his two previously published essays: "Caregiving: The Odyssey of Becoming More Human," *The Lancet* 373, no. 9660 (2009): 292–93 and "Catastrophe and Caregiving: The Failure of Medicine as an Art," *The Lancet* 371, no. 9606 (2008): 22–23.

3. See, for example, Paul Farmer et al., eds., *Women, Poverty, and AIDS: Sex, Drugs, and Structural Violence* (Monroe, Maine: Common Courage Press, 1996).

4. Jim Yong Kim et al., "From a Declaration of Values to the Creation of Value in Global Health: A Report from Harvard University's Global Health Delivery Project," *Global Public Health* 5, no. 2 (2010): 181–8.

5. MVA is a medical acronym for a motor vehicle accident.

6. Countway Library is the principal library associated with Harvard Medical School.

7. OSHA is the Occupational Safety and Health Administration, a federal agency charged with implementing laws concerning health and safety. OSHA reports are not known for brevity.

8. Dr. Joseph Martin served as Dean of the Harvard Faculty of Medicine from 1997 to 2007.

9. HST refers to the Health Sciences and Technology program, a joint Harvard-MIT medical school track that is oriented toward students with an interest in biomedical research and a background in physical or biological sciences.

10. Jonas Salk was an American medical researcher best known for discovering and developing the first polio vaccine in 1955. Soon after, Albert Sabin developed an attenuated oral polio vaccine that was used to vaccinate millions of people. Louis Pasteur was a French microbiologist whose experiments helped establish the germ theory of disease. Pasteur also developed the first vaccine for rabies in 1885 and came up with the process of treating milk (pasteurization) to prevent the spread of disease.

11. Martin Luther King Jr., speech given at the Second National Convention of the Medical Committee for Human Rights, Chicago, IL (March 25, 1966).

12. "The Economics of Empire: Notes on the Washington Consensus," *Harper's Magazine*, May, 2003.

13. The "Second-year Show" is an annual comic play put on by second-year students at Harvard Medical School.

14. Carl Hiaasen, *Skin Tight* (New York: Berkley Books, 1989), 11.

15. Ibid., chap. 30.

16. Associated Press, "Calusas May Have Fled to Cuba," *Miami Herald* (March 15, 2004).

17. Eve Kerr et al., "Profiling the Quality of Care in Twelve Com-

munities: Results from the CQI Study," *Health Affairs* 23, no. 3 (May 2004).

18. Donna Shalala, a professor of political science and education and former Secretary of Health and Human Services under President Bill Clinton, has served as president of the University of Miami since 2001.

19. Brigham and Women's Hospital in Boston; Paul Farmer serves as Chief of the Division of Global Health Equity.

20. For more on Haiti's history, see Paul Farmer, *The Uses of Haiti* (Monroe, ME: Common Courage Press, 1994).

21. Boston Children's Hospital and Massachusetts General Hospital are Harvard-affiliated hospitals in Boston.

22. P. Lawrence et al., "The Water Poverty Index: An International Comparison," *Keele Economic Research Papers* (2002); see also the 2008 report by the Center for Human Rights and Global Justice and the Global Justice Clinic at New York University's School of Law, Partners In Health, Zanmi Lasante, and the Robert F. Kennedy Center for Justice and Human Rights "Wòch nan Soley: The Denial of the Right to Water in Haiti," www.pih.org/page/-/reports/Haiti_Report_FINAL.pdf.

23. Official estimates of the death toll of the 2010 earthquake range from 220,000 to 316,000. For more on the complexities associated with making such estimates, see Farmer, *Haiti After the Earthquake*, 119.

24. IRBs stands for institutional review boards, regulatory bodies charged with reviewing the ethical implications of proposed research involving human subjects.

25. Bascom-Palmer Eye Institute is the ophthalmic care center at the University of Miami Leonard M. Miller School of Medicine.

PART III: HEALTH, HUMAN RIGHTS, AND UNNATURAL DISASTERS

1. Quoted in Theodore M. Brown and Elizabeth Fee, "Rudolph Carl Virchow: Medical Scientist, Social Reformer, Role Model," *American Journal of Public Health* (December 2006) 96: 2104.

2. The Nurses' Health Study was launched in 1976 to track the potential long-term consequences of oral contraceptive use among nurses. The cohort study, renewed in 1989 and again in 2010, has gathered data from more than 238,000 participants about how a range of lifestyle factors affect health outcomes. The Physicians' Health Study was a randomized trial established in 1982 to track the effects of aspirin in the prevention of cardiovascular disease and cancer among physicians. A second trial was established in 1997 to test the risks and benefits of vitamins C, E, and a multivitamin.

3. Barry Bloom, an expert in infectious disease research, served as dean of the Harvard School of Public Health from 1998 to 2008.

4. James K. Galbraith, "A Perfect Crime: Inequality in the Age of Globalization," *Daedalus* (Winter 2002), 22.

5. NICU is a medical acronym for neonatal intensive care unit.

6. Steven L. Gortmaker and Paul H. Wise, "The First Injustice: Socioeconomic Disparities, Health Services Technology, and Infant Mortality," *Annual Review of Sociology* 23 (1997): 147–70.

7. Peter Vinten-Johansen et al., *Cholera, Chloroform, and the Science of Medicine: A Life of John Snow* (New York: Oxford University Press, 2003), 7.

8. Vinten-Johansen et al., 7.

9. Ackerknecht, Erwin, *Rudolph Virchow: Doctor, Statesman, Anthropologist* (Madison: University of Wisconsin Press, 1953).

10. Bertolt Brecht, "A Worker's Speech to a Doctor" ("Rede eines Arbeiters an einen Arzt," *Spätere Gedichte und Satiren aus Svendborg,* 1936–38), in *The Body in the Library: A Literary Anthology of Modern Medicine,* ed. Iain Bamforth, (London: Verso, 2003), 167–68.

11. Howard Hiatt, *Medical Lifeboat: Will There Be Room for You in the Health Care System?* (New York: Harper & Row, 1987), ix.

12. Save the Children, *State of the World's Mother 2006: Saving the Lives of Mothers and Newborns* (Westport, CT: Save the Children, 2006).

13. Paul Krugman, "Our Sick Society," *New York Times* (May 5, 2006), A26.

14. R.D. Moore et al., "Racial Differences in the Use of Drug Therapy for HIV Disease in an Urban Community," *New England Journal of Medicine* 330 (1994): 763–68.

15. S.B. Lucas et al., "The Mortality and Pathology of HIV Infection in a West African City," *AIDS* 7 (1993): 1569–79.

16. R.E. Chaisson, J.C. Keruly, and R.D. Moore, "Race, Sex, Drug Use, and Progression of Human Immunodeficiency Virus Disease," *New England Journal of Medicine* 333 (1995): 751–56.

17. Richard Rhodes, *The Making of the Atomic Bomb* (New York: Touchstone, 1986), 490.

18. Benjamin Sachs, an obstetrician and expert in reducing medical errors, has served as dean of the Tulane School of Medicine since 2007.

19. *Hoya Saxa* is the official cheer of Georgetown University. *Hoya* is an Ancient Greek word *hoios*, meaning "such a" or "what a," while *saxa* is Latin for "rocks." The complete phrase is often translated as "what rocks!" Over the last century and despite its ambiguous origins, *Hoya* has become the proud nickname for Georgetown's athletic teams and students. See http://alumni.georgetown.edu/ccg/ccg_17.html.

20. Steven Johnson, *Where Good Ideas Come From: A Natural History of Innovation* (New York: Riverhead, 2010), 31.

21. Adam Gopnik, "How the Internet Gets Inside Us," the *New Yorker*, February 14, 2011.

22. Martin Luther King Jr., "Beyond Vietnam," speech delivered April 4, 1967, at Riverside Church, New York.

23. See also "Accompaniment as Policy," Kennedy School of Government Commencement Speech 2011, in this volume.

24. Bill Clinton, *Giving: How Each of Us Can Change the World* (New York: Knopf, 2007), 207.

25. Ibid., x.

26. Ibid., 3.

27. See Paul Farmer, "Countering Failures of Imagination," Northwestern University Commencement Speech 2012, in this volume.

PART IV: SERVICE, SOLIDARITY, SOCIAL JUSTICE

1. The Union Medal was awarded jointly to Paul Farmer and Ophelia Dahl, two of the five cofounders of Partners In Health.

2. Dietrich Bonhoeffer, "After Ten Years: A Reckoning Made at New Year 1943," in *Letters and Papers from Prison*, ed. Eberhand Bethge

(New York: Macmillan, 1967), 17. "After Ten Years" acquired a new, final paragraph in the 1970 edition of *Letters and Papers*. Eberhard Bethge, Bonhoeffer's friend and editor and himself a former Union medalist, believed this paragraph was unfinished but was intended to close the reckoning. If so, it's a simple peroration, an incomplete gesture. But it mattered to Bonhoeffer and to those who knew him best.

3. Interview on National Public Radio with Juan Williams, "Secretary Colin L. Powell," Washington, DC (March 8, 2004), http://2001-2009.state.gov/secretary/former/powell/remarks/30245.htm.

4. Bonhoeffer, 4.

5. See Paul Farmer, "Pestilence and Restraint: Guantánamo, AIDS, and the Logic of Quarantine," in *Pathologies of Power: Health, Human Rights, and the New War on the Poor* (Berkeley: University of California Press, 2003), 51–90.

6. A. Schoenholtz, "Aiding and Abetting Persecutors: The Seizure and Return of Haitian Refugees in Violation of the U.N. Refugee Convention and Protocol," *Georgetown Immigration Law Journal* 7, no. 1 (1993): 67–85.

7. Cited in G.J. Annas, "Detention of HIV-positive Haitians at Guantánamo: Human Rights and Medical Care," *New England Journal of Medicine* 329, no. 8 (1993): 589–92.

8. See Farmer, "Pestilence and Restraint."

9. Jim Michaels, "Behind Success in Ramadi: An Army Colonel's Gamble," *USA Today* (May 1, 2007), 1–2.

10. Jonathan Hansen, "Guantánamo: An American Story," lecture given at Harvard University (April 26, 2007). See also Hansen's recent book *Guantánamo: An American History* (New York: Hill and Wang, 2011).

11. Marcus Tullius Cicero, *M. Tulli Ciceronis ad. M. Brutum Orator*, translated by Sir John Edwin Sandys, (London: Cambridge University Press, 1885).

12. Susan Sontag, *Regarding the Pain of Others* (New York: Farrar, Strauss, and Giroux, 2003), 114.

13. "Harper's Index," *Harper's Magazine,* May 2007, 13.

14. Cited in Richard Dawkins, *The God Delusion* (London: Bantam Press, 2006), 15.

15. Ibid.

16. Jim Wallis, *The Great Awakening: Reviving Faith and Politics in a Post-Religious Right America* (New York: HarperOne, 2008), 25.

17. Wallis, 12.

18. Each year, some 20,000 alumni and their families attend Reunion and Commencement weekend activities at Princeton University. Fireworks follow the annual, public, and well-loved University Orchestra evening lawn concert. See "Nassau Notes," *Princeton Weekly Bulletin*, May 19, 2008, 27, http://www.princeton.edu/pr/pwb/08/0519/nn/.

19. Seamus Heaney, *The Cure at Troy: A Version of Sophocles' Philoctetes* (New York: Farrar, Straus and Giroux, 1991), 77.

20. "Nixon's Nose" is the affectionate nickname for Henry Moore's iconic sculpture, *Oval with Points*, positioned by West College on the Princeton campus. See the *Daily Princetonian*, October 6, 1999, 8. Princeton is also home to 11 historic private eating clubs, which are an important part of social and nutritional life on campus. See http://www.princeton.edu/main/campuslife/housingdining/eatingclubs/.

21. Martin Luther King Jr., *Where Do We Go from Here: Chaos or Community?* (New York: Harper & Row, 1967).

22. Martin Luther King Jr., Presentation at the Second National Convention of the Medical Committee for Human Rights, Chicago, IL (March 25, 1966).

23. Martin Luther King Jr., "The Casualties of the War in Vietnam," The Nation Institute, Los Angeles, CA (February 25, 1967).

24. Martin Luther King Jr., *Where Do We Go from Here?*

25. Martin Luther King Jr., "Beyond Vietnam: A Time to Break Silence," speech delivered at a meeting of Clergy and Laity Concerned About Vietnam at Riverside Church in New York City (April 4, 1967).

26. Editorial, *Life*, April 21, 1967.

27. "A Tragedy," the *Washington Post*, April 1967, A20.

28. Martin Luther King Jr., "Remaining Awake Through a Great Revolution," Oberlin College Commencement Speech (June 14, 1965).

29. Martin Luther King Jr., "Beyond Vietnam," speech delivered April 4, 1967, at Riverside Church, New York.

30. Martin Luther King Jr., *Where Do We Go from Here?*

31. Martin Luther King Jr., "The Drum Major Instinct," sermon delivered at Ebenezer Baptist Church, Atlanta, GA (February 4, 1968).

32. Rudolf Virchow, "Der Armenartzt," cited in Erwin Heinz Ackerknecht, *Rudolf Virchow: Doctor, Statesman, Anthropologist* (Madison: University of Wisconsin Press, 1953), 46.

33. Paul Farmer et al., "Tuberculosis, Poverty, and 'Compliance': Lessons from Rural Haiti," *Seminars in Respiratory Infections* 6, no. 4 (1991): 254–60.

34. Carole Mitnick et al., "Community-based Therapy for Multidrug-resistant Tuberculosis in Lima, Peru," *New England Journal of Medicine* 348, no. 2 (2003).

35. H. L. Behforouz, Paul Farmer, and J. S. Mukherjee, "From Directly Observed Therapy to *Accompagnateurs*: Enhancing Aids Treatment Outcomes in Haiti and in Boston," *Clinical Infectious Diseases* 38, Suppl 5 (2004): S429–36.

36. Eric Larsen and Daniel Pederson, "Too Poor to Treat," *Newsweek,* July 27, 2007.

37. Paul Farmer et al., "Community-based Approaches to HIV Treatment in Resource-poor Settings," *Lancet* 358, no. 9279 (2001): 404–409.

38. For more on the etymology of *accompaniment*, see Roberto Goizueta, *Caminemos con Jesus: Toward a Hispanic/Latino Theology of Accompaniment* (Maryknoll, NY: Orbis Books, 2003).

39. See, e.g., Gustavo Guitiérrez, *The Power of the Poor in History: Selected Writings* (Maryknoll, NY: Orbis Books, 1973).

40. Goizueta, *Caminemos*, 192.

41. Goizueta, *Caminemos*, 199. The distances are not only spatial but temporal. It may be possible to accompany those who have already suffered and died. The first class I taught at Harvard was as my mentor's teaching fellow. Arthur Kleinman and I taught a course we designed together and called it, *à la* William James, "Varieties of Human Suffering." We showed Claude Lanzmann's film, *Shoah*. I was recently reminded that, for the filmmaker, the most "profound" and "incomprehensible" part about the experience of making the film was a sense of accompanying "all those who died alone." In an essay called "*Shoah* as Shivah," historian Michael Roth picks up on this point: "In accompa-

nying these people, in passing with them through the past, Lanzmann performs what Jewish law calls a 'highly meritorious act.' He comes to dwell with those who suffer loss, and with some who are lost in their suffering. The absence is to be made present for the community of mourners through a ritual that brings the dead to mind, to voice." Michael Roth, "*Shoah* as Shivah," *The Ironist's Cage: Memory, Trauma and the Construction of History* (New York: Columbia University Press, 1995), 225–26.

42. United Nations Office of the Special Envoy for Haiti, "Has Aid Changed? Channelling Assistance to Haiti before and after the Earthquake," June 2011, http://www.haitispecialenvoy.org/download/ Report_Center/has_aid_changed_en.pdf.

43. These numbers are, of course, contested. For an overview of both contradictory numbers and their origins, see Paul Farmer, *Haiti After the Earthquake* (New York: PublicAffairs Books, 2011), 118–20.

44. Martha Mendoza, "Would-be Haitian Contractors Miss Out on Aid," Associated Press (December 12, 2010), http://news.yahoo.com/s/ ap/20101212/ap_on_re_us/cb_haiti_outsourcing_aid_1.

45. Isabelle Defourny et al., "Management of Moderate Acute Malnutrition with RUTF in Niger," *MSF Report* (2007), http://www.msf .org.au/uploads/media/mod_acc_mal_Niger.pdf.

46. Of course there have been sharp disagreements about this matter, including the question of whether or not RUTF, this miraculous treatment for malnutrition, should be subject to international patent law. See, for example, Andrew Rice's exposé "The Peanut Solution" in the *New York Times Magazine,* September 2, 2010, http://www.nytimes .com/2010/09/05/magazine/05plumpy-t.html?pagewanted=all. We're confident that the accompaniment approach will lead many partners away from ready acquiescence to intellectual property regimes that make sense for some therapeutics but not others.

47. This example is discussed at length in Farmer, *Haiti After the Earthquake.*

48. Malcolm Gladwell, "Creation Myth," the *New Yorker,* May 16, 2011, 50.

49. Atul Gawande, *The Checklist Manifesto: How to Get Things Right* (New York: Metropolitan Books, 2009).

50. Mercedes Becerra et al., "Using Treatment Failure under Effective Directly Observed Short-Course Chemotherapy Programs to Identify Patients with Multidrug-resistant Tuberculosis," *International Journal of Tuberculosis and Lung Disease* 4, no. 2 (2000): 108–14.

51. The historian Michael Roth has observed: "The privileging of irony is often the result of the inability to sustain belief in the possibilities of significant political change" (p. 148). His book about memory, trauma, and the construction of history is titled, with a nod to Weber, *The Ironist's Cage.*

52. As Bill Clinton notes, "Many of the problems that bedevil both rich and poor nations in the modern world cannot be adequately addressed without more enlightened government policies, more competent and honest public administration, and more investment of tax dollars. There is plenty of evidence that more effective government can produce higher incomes, better living conditions, more social justice, and a cleaner environment across the board. But in many areas, regardless of the quality of government, a critical difference is being made by citizens working as individuals, in businesses, and through nongovernmental, nonprofit organizations." Bill Clinton, *Giving: How Each of Us Can Change the World* (New York: Random House, 2007), 4.

ACKNOWLEDGMENTS

In the acknowledgments of previous books, Paul has tried to thank some of the TNTC—too numerous to count—people who have helped grow the work of Partners In Health from its humble beginnings in central Haiti in 1983. To avoid repetition, we will keep this short, even though many have contributed to these speeches and to this volume.

First, we'd like to thank Naomi Schneider and her team at University of California Press, who believed in this book from the beginning. We are grateful to Haun Saussy, Paul's lifelong editor-in-chief, who over the years went through just about every one of these speeches with a fine-toothed comb. We're also indebted to Chelsea Clinton for her invaluable contributions to the manuscript.

Second, we'd like to thank all of Paul's hosts and accompagnateurs. Paul wouldn't have gotten far—much less to the podium on time—without them. Special thanks go to those accompagnateurs-in-chief, the McCormack family, and also to Laurie

Nuell and her sister to whom this book is dedicated; they remind us always of the "ministry of showing up."

Finally, our greatest thanks are reserved for the extraordinary team at Partners In Health, Harvard Medical School, and Brigham and Women's Hospital who, in the words of Jen Puccetti, "keep the trains running." In particular, we are grateful to David Walton, Cynthia Rose, Melissa Gillooly, Naomi Rosenberg, Alice Yang, Cassia van der Hoof Holstein, Matt Basilico, Luke Messac, Zoe Agoos, Emily Bahnsen, Jon Niconchuk, Gretchen Williams, Mary Block, Kevin Savage, and Vicky Koski-Karell for their assistance over the years in bringing these speeches and this volume into being.

These are just a few of the people who deserve mention for their tireless efforts to help "repair the world," as our perhaps overly grand title puts it. Our deepest thanks to all those who make this work possible.